Be

a

Baby

How Your Unborn Baby Grows from Day-to-Day

by

William F. Supple, Jr., Ph. D.

Becoming a Baby

Supple, William F. Jr., Ph. D.
Becoming a baby - How your unborn baby grows from day-to-day.
/ W. F. Supple, Jr.
p. 288 cm.
Includes references and index.
ISBN 0-96539-114-0
1. Pregnancy - popular works 2. Fetal development
3. Pregnancy

Picket Fence Publishing
South Burlington, Vermont USA

http://www.BecomingaBaby.com

Printed in Canada

This book is not intended to be used as a substitute for competent medical advice. Adhere to the advice and recommendations of your health care provider.

To Dorothy Goddard Patterson (1913 - 2002)
A true Renaissance woman with an active and full mind,
prepared and equipped to challenge traditional ideas.
You will be greatly missed.

*****

Acknowledgments - The images contained in this book are available due to the gracious generosity of the authors listed below and their publishers. We deeply appreciate their assistance by allowing us the privilege of using their fine works.

Streeter, G. L. (1951). Developmental horizons in human embryos. Carnegie Institute of Washington, Washington D.C. Images from Day 10-12, 25-28, 30-48, 50-56, 58, 59 modified.

Kretztechunk AG, Medison Corporation. Images from Day 55, 60, 64, 67, 70, 75, 80, 91, 105, 107, 108, 123, 126, 138, 139, 140, 150-152, 154, 160, 164-167, 173-175, 179, 183, 187, 189, 191, 192, 195, 196, 200-206, 209-212, 214-218, 220, 221, 226, 227, 229-231, 234-236, 243, 245, 246, 248-262, 264, 265 modified.

Moore, K. L., Persaud, T.V.N., & Shiota, K (1994). Color atlas of clinical embryology. WB Saunders: New York. Images from Day 8-9, 14-24, 62-66, 68, 69, 71-74, 76-79, 81-84, 87-90, 92, 95, 96, 98. 100, 101, 106, 109-112, 114-118, 120-122, 124, 125, 127-137, 142-146, 148, 149, 155, 159, 161,162, 163, 166, 168, 171, 172, 176-178, 180, 184, 186, 188, 190, 219, 222, 223 modified.

England, M. (1996). Life before birth. Mosby: London. Images from Day 103, 104, 233, 242 modified.

University of Michigan Health Sciences. Images from Day 29, 57, 85, 113, 141, 169, 197 and 225 modified.

This book is designed for expectant parents as an easy-to-use guide to take you through all the major developmental milestones that happen during the next 266 days (38 weeks) culminating in the birth of your child. This fetal development calendar provides a day-by-day account of the changes in your child as it progresses through the embryonic and fetal stages. Facts about the baby are indicated by the baby image shown. You will learn when your baby's bones begin to appear and when fingernails form, when it can hear and kick, what it can sense and perceive, learn and remember.

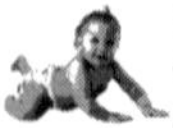

Included also are physiological and psychological changes the mother may experience at each stage of pregnancy. As a place marker, this 'pregnant woman' image indicates the passage presenting information about the mother.

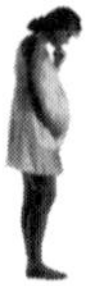

The development of your baby is organized into lunar months each consisting of 28 days, with four weeks per month. The developmental events described are synchronized with the moment of conception, and continue each day until birth 266 days later.

The calendar starts at conception or fertilization, which is probably a few weeks earlier than when you received this calendar. Therefore, you may want to read through the 2 or 3 weeks that your baby has progressed up to your current Day of pregnancy. To help accurately determine the prenatal age of your unborn baby, you can visit http://www.BecomingaBaby.com. You'll find a 'prenatal age calculator' that will help you.

As you'll see, not every day contains a noticeable external change in your baby but that's part of the miracle of development. I tried to present the most important information without getting bogged down in too much detail. References are given for further reading where you can explore a topic in detail.

You'll have many questions flash through your mind that you'll want to ask your health care provider. Take this book with you to your visits. Most pages have a space to jot down questions so that you'll be reminded what to ask at each appointment. Also write down the suggestions or advice given to you by your doctor, nurse or midwife.

. My writing this calendar was inspired by the experiences my wife and I had prior to the birth of our first daughter, Anna. We were curious about her day-to-day development from the very start, wondering what she looked like each day and how she was growing. We quickly learned that the questions we had were not answered in most of the books commonly available. We wanted to know what was going on with our baby now...today. We found ourselves consulting primary medical textbooks to view pictures of babies at various stages of development to satisfy our curiosity.

My training as a behavioral neuroscientist helped me to research the range and complexity of behaviors shown by these unborn babies at the very earliest stages of development. Unlike earlier ideas of the unborn as 'witless tadpoles,' I have come to appreciate the sophistication of the behavior shown by developing babies. Unborn babies are behaving, reacting, learning beings whose abilities are just starting to be appreciated. What I have realized in the course of this work is that unborn babies are clearly more advanced than we commonly believe and that they will be shown, over time, to be very capable and behaviorally complex, much earlier than ever imagined. The tools to discover many of these fascinating behaviors have yet to be invented. As you progress through this book you will see that a baby is a very competent being adapted to the aquatic environment of the womb and forced to adapt to a terrestrial environment after birth. This change in environment contributes to the apparent helplessness of the newborn.

I wish to thank my wife, Toni, for her helpful editing and content suggestions that have made this calendar more 'user-friendly' and clear.

I hope this calendar answers some of the questions that arise each and every day during the course of your pregnancy and enhances the excitement that accompanies these very special days leading up to the birth of your new child.

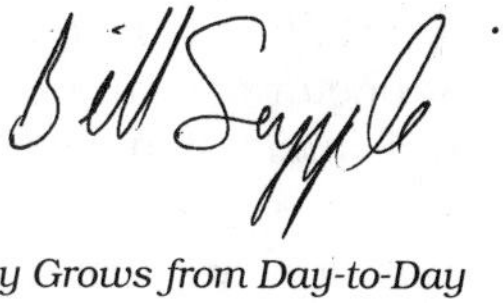

How to use this fetal development calendar.

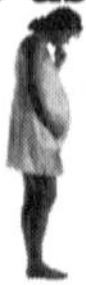

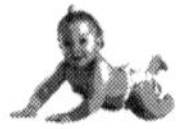

This book presents the day-by-day changes that occur in your developing baby. The calendar starts at Day 1, which marks the day of conception which is the start of the developmental period for your baby. There are 266 days that mark the usual gestation or development period for a baby. Since you will probably start reading this book sometime after conception, you may not have a good idea of when Day 1 actually was for your baby. You have a few options to estimate the actual date of Day 1. First, when your health care provider determines your due date, you can count backwards to try to determine when conception may have occurred. Second, you may remember the actual day conception occurred. Or third, you could take your best guess and estimate the day of conception. It really doesn't matter whether your pregnancy is exactly synchronized with the calendar, you'll be close enough to the actual progress of your baby whether you estimate the day of conception or know the day for sure. You may also wish to visit http://www.BecomingaBaby.com, enter some simple information and determine the exact prenatal age of your baby!

Your doctor or health care provider will count the days and weeks of your pregnancy differently than this calendar. The time course of pregnancy includes the two weeks before conception - dating back to the first day of your last menstrual period. So your doctor's references to your pregnancy, for example, that you're 12 weeks pregnant, means that your baby is actually in the 10th week of gestation. Just remember that your doctor's reference to the stage of your pregnancy will be 2 weeks ahead of the actual gestational week of your baby's development. So, as an example, if on May 1 your doctor determines that you are 10 weeks pregnant the day of conception was March 6 - eight weeks earlier.

DAY 1

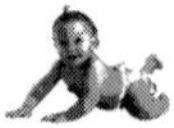

He who sees things grow from the beginning will have the finest view of them -- *Aristotle, Greek philosopher, 384-322 B.C.*

The first day of pregnancy is the day fertilization occurs. One lucky sperm out of about 350 million will penetrate the egg and start the process of development The successful sperm embeds within the outside covering of the egg, releases enzymes to dissolve an opening, and enters. Half of the genetic information (DNA) is provided by the egg, the other half is provided by the father's sperm. Fertilization usually occurs in the fallopian tube shortly after the egg is released by the ovary.

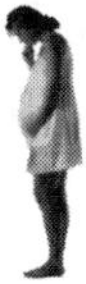

A healthy diet will soon pay off because much of the early development of the baby occurs before you realize that you're pregnant.

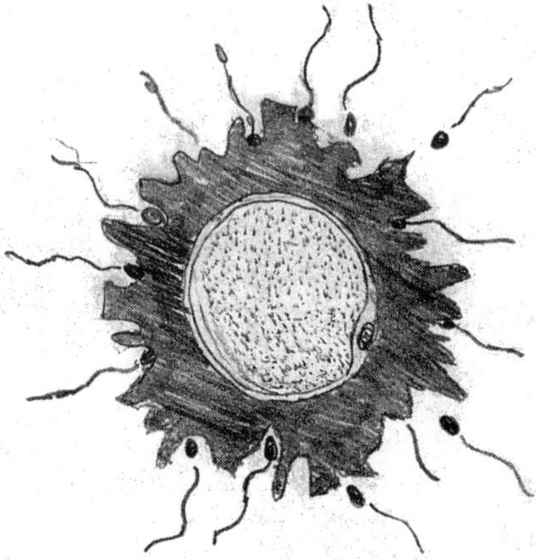

Notes:

....

....

DAY 2

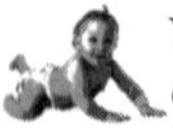

Whether you have a boy or a girl is already decided! The sex of the child is determined by the father's sperm. There are two types of sperm: X or Y, produced in equal numbers. If a Y sperm fertilizes the egg, a boy results; if an X reaches a girl results. Some behavioral differences have been noted between X and Y sperm. Y sperm are faster swimmers but die sooner; X sperm are slower but live longer.

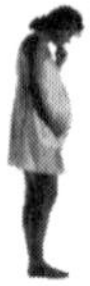

Remember that what you eat your baby eats. This includes various substances that could have an adverse effect on the baby. For example, when you ingest drugs like caffeine or alcohol it crosses through the placenta and affects the baby the same way it affects you.

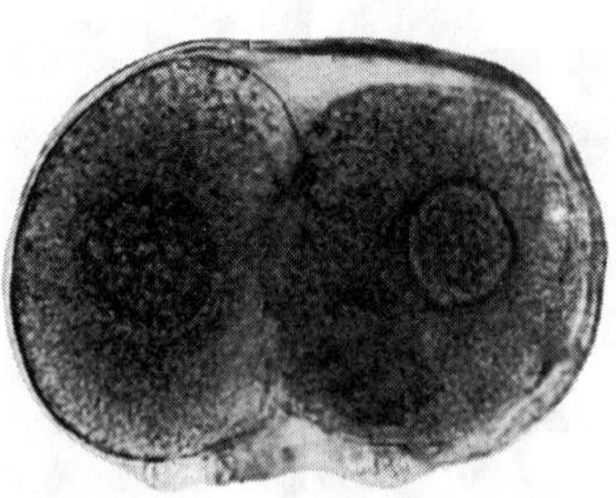

Two cell zygote (fertilized egg)

Thoughts:

....

....

DAY 3

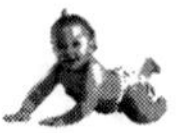

As the fertilized egg makes its way through the fallopian tube it will start to change. Increases in the number of cells will occur by cell division, resulting in a hollow ball of 16 cells shaped like a mulberry as it enters the top of the uterus from the fallopian tube. In fact, the name for the group of cells at this stage is morula, which means mulberry in Latin.

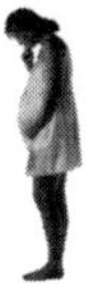

Folic acid -- Vitamin B_9 -- has been shown to be important in the prevention of certain birth defects. Folic acid is commonly added to "fortified" cereals and breads. Other sources are dark green leafy vegetables, citrus fruits and beans. Many broad-range supplemental vitamins also have folic acid. Most doctors recommend between 600 - 800 micrograms of folic acid per day.

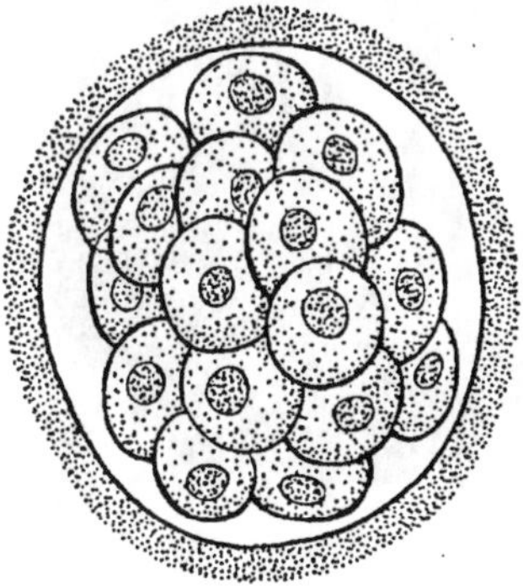

Notes:

....

....

DAY 4

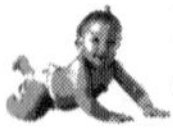

Development is now at a stage where the cells take the form of a ball of cells (early blastocyst) - let's call it baby blastula. From here these few cells will change (differentiate) into the various parts and organ systems of the body. Baby blastula is a hollow ball of 68 cells with a fluid center. It is still traveling through the fallopian tube.

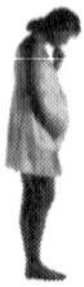

Smoking can reduce the birth weight of babies. A recent study found that the risk of having an underweight baby increased with the number of cigarettes smoked per day. If you smoke now, quit. Every cigarette that you don't smoke is one less cigarette that your baby will smoke.

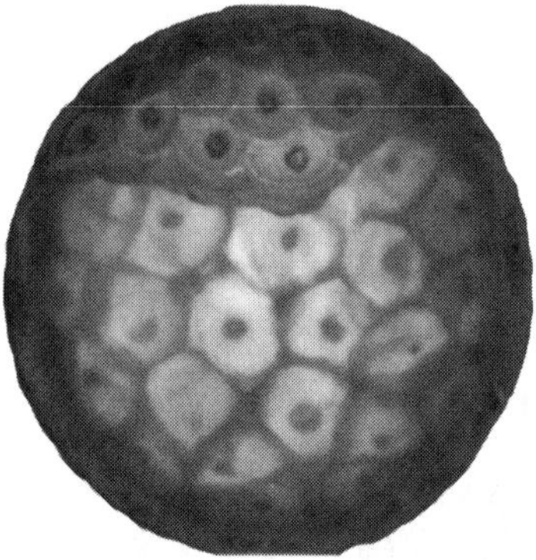

Thoughts:

....

....

DAY 5

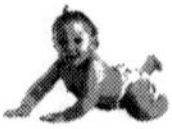

Baby blastula has changed shape and size, increasing to 107 cells, and is preparing to implant itself in the wall of the uterus when it arrives there tomorrow.

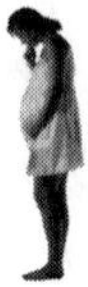

The cells at this point could be mistaken for a potentially dangerous invader like a bacteria or virus. There is a substance released called Early Pregnancy Factor that blocks the mother's reaction to the developing cells, enabling the pregnancy to continue.

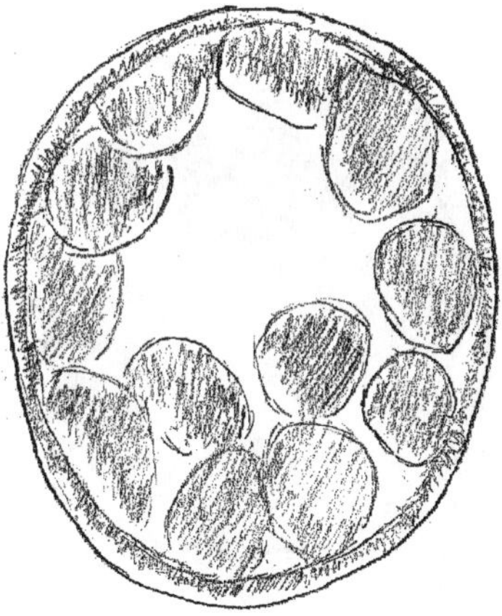

Notes:

....

....

DAY 6

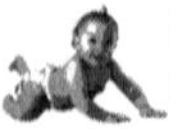

Baby blastula now begins the process of implantation into the lining of the uterus. Over the course of the next few days, the foundation for the blood supply to the embryo will develop into the forerunner of the placenta.

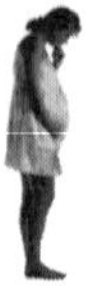

Progesterone is a hormone now present that helps maintain your pregnancy...progesterone literally means facilitating gestation (development). Progesterone is manufactured by the pituitary gland at the base of the mother's brain. Later on in the pregnancy, the developing placenta will be a major source of the progesterone needed to support and maintain your baby.

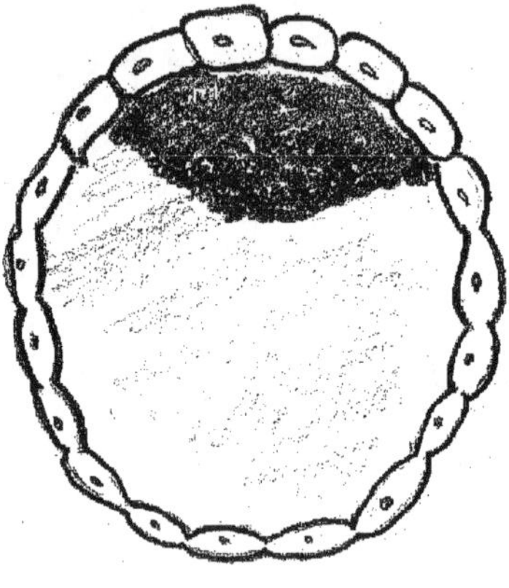

Thoughts:

....

....

DAY 7

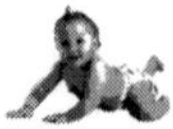

Baby blastula more firmly attaches itself to the uterine wall (endometrium) and blood vessel connections start to form. This connection between the endometrium and baby blastula is where the placenta will form.

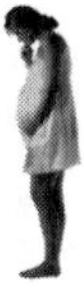

You might expect equal numbers of boys and girls to be born because X and Y sperms are formed in equal numbers. However, there are more boys born in all countries and in the United States there are 105 boys born to every 100 girls born. There is no widely accepted scientific explanation for this difference in sex ratio. Smoking does decrease the male babies born. The male-to-female ratio is 1.21 among parents who never smoked (1.21 males born for every female born). Whereas among parents that both smoked greater than 20 cigarettes/day the ratio was .82 (.82 males born for every female). Even if the mother didn't smoke, a father who smoked more than 20 cigarettes/day reduced the odds of a male to .98.

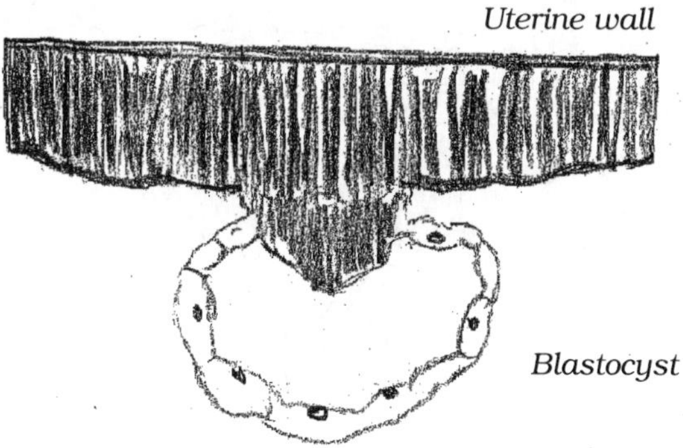

Notes:

....

....

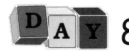

DAY 8

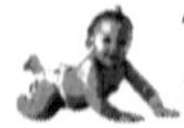

The part of the womb where baby blastula is most likely to implant is in the middle of the uterus on the back wall. Almost all implantations occur very close to a maternal capillary, suggesting that there is some sort of attractive factor toward maternal blood that influences where baby blastula attaches to the uterus. The closer to a source of blood, the easier it should be to develop connections between the baby and the mother through the later forming placenta.

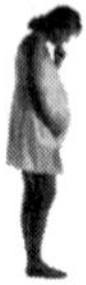

Some women are fooled into thinking they aren't pregnant by what is known as 'implantation bleeding.' This is a small amount of blood that may be shed as a result of the baby blastocyst's implantation. The blood can be mistaken as the beginning of a period.

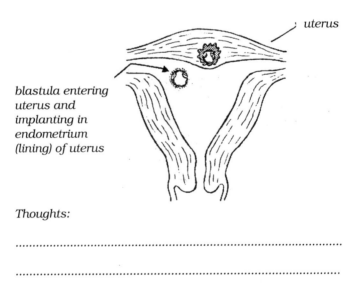

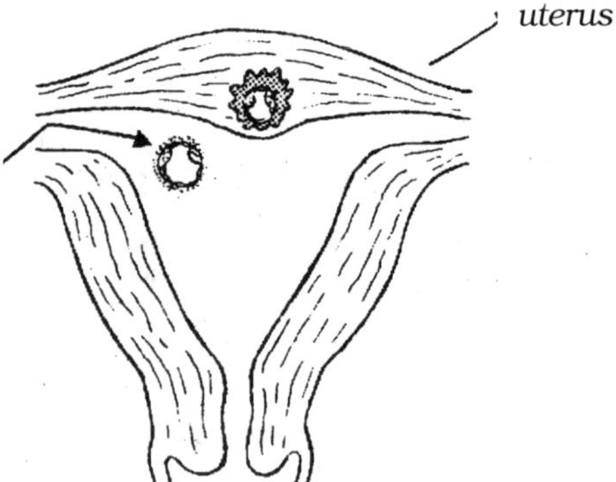

Thoughts:

....

....

DAY 9

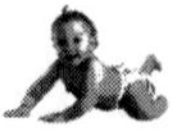

Baby blastula continues to develop rich vascular connections with the uterine wall in preparation for the phenomenal growth that will soon occur. A hint of our link to other animals is shown by the appearance of a primitive yolk sac that will disappear soon.

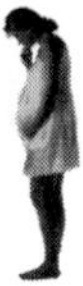

Twins - About 1 out of 40 pregnancies involves twins. Identical twins are also called monozygotic twins because they come from the same egg and contain the exact same genetic information. Twinning takes place around this day as implantation is progressing. Identical twins share one placenta but each baby will be encased in its own amnionic sac.

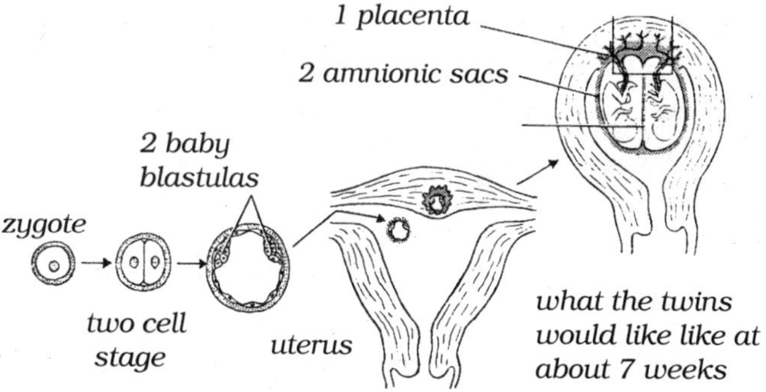

Notes:

....

....

DAY 10

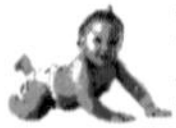

Baby blastula is now completely implanted, actually sinking below the surface of the endometrium. The beginnings of a placenta will start to form in the next few days. The amniotic sac, which will contain amniotic fluid, will start to form.

Development progresses from relatively simple to more complex. Embryos from other species are similar early on and then differentiate and take on their unique species-typical appearance during the fetal stage.

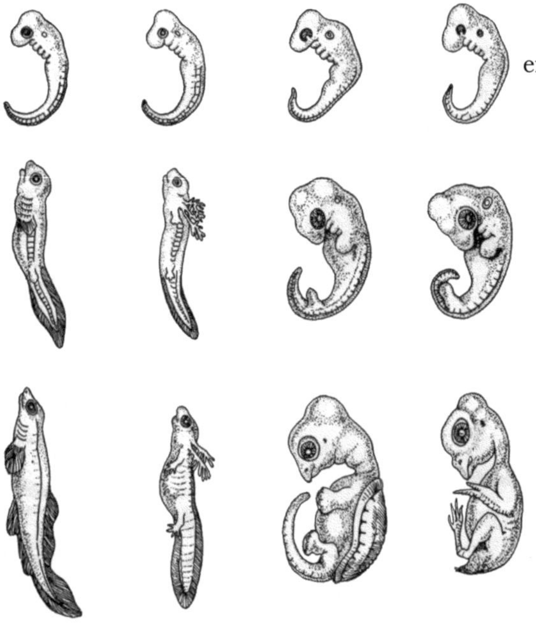

DAY 11

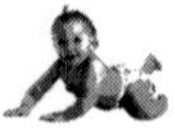

Connections start to form that will become the placental circulatory system, to exchange nutrients, water and waste products between the mother and her baby. Baby blastula now has a new name : embryo. The embryo is still very small, measuring only one-fifth of a millimeter, still too small to be seen easily with the naked eye.

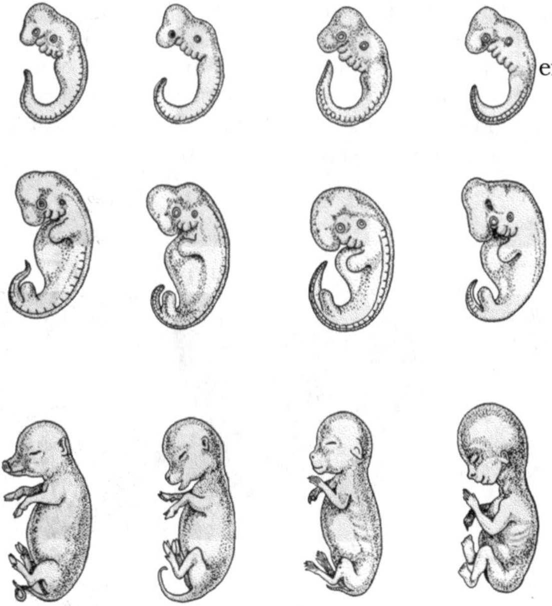

DAY 12

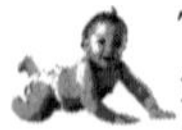

The placenta continues to form with maternal blood seeping into regions around the embryo, and the start of an early circulatory system between the uterus and placenta takes root. Until the placenta is functioning, the embryo will get its nutrition and energy for growth from the contents of the yolk sac.

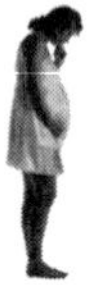

Due Dates: The estimation of when your baby will be born is really more of an educated guess. Only 4% of all babies are delivered on the exact due date assigned by your health care professional. Part of the variability has to do with determining when to start counting days. Whether the day of conception/fertilization is used or the date of the last menstrual period (and then counting backwards two weeks) is used, both figures involve some inherent uncertainty. A larger factor is that babies are responsible for the initiation of labor based on the release of a chemical 'signal.' When and how that signal is released is unknown.

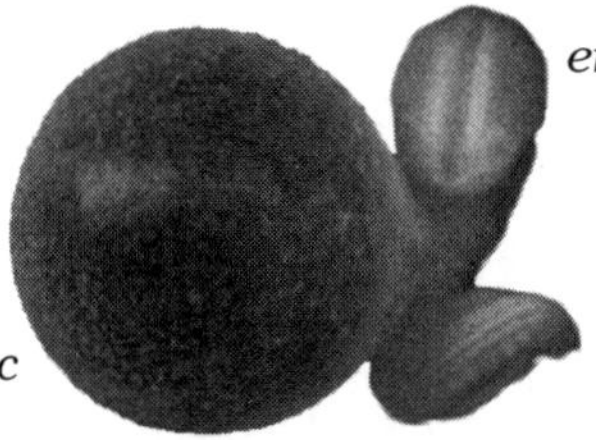

Thoughts:

....

....

DAY 13

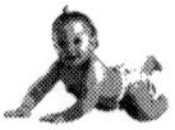

The outer covering of the sac enclosing the embryo, known as the chorionic villi, is growing fast. This growth increases the levels of hCG hormone in your blood which is what will register on the pregnancy test. While it is still too early to detect pregnancy with chemical (urine) tests, ultrasound tests could locate the embryo now.

The cardiovascular system starts to develop with blood vessels starting to form. The embryo's heart will start beating in one week.

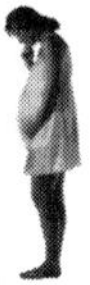

Zinc is an essential trace element necessary for the development of bone, and is involved in growth (protein synthesis). Not many foods - other than oysters - contain zinc...20 mg per day is the recommended amount during pregnancy. Your supplemental vitamin should have zinc.

Hormone levels will start to change rapidly in your body now that baby blastula is implanted in the uterus. The hormonal changes include increased levels of progesterone, human chorionic gonadotrophin (hCG) and estrogen. These hormones are necessary to sustain the pregnancy. However, the levels of these hormones (most notably hCG) is still to faint to detect with standard hormone-detecting pregnancy tests. The hormone hCG is produced by baby blastula and excreted in your urine in small amounts. In about a week you'll know for sure that you're pregnant because that's when the over-the-counter home tests will start to work.

Notes:

....

....

DAY 14

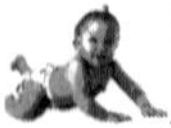

First missed menstrual period...somethings up!

Vascularization between the embryo and mother continues with an increase in the amount of amniotic fluid.

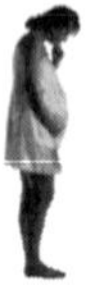

Room for expansion: The size of your uterus will expand from that of the volume of a grape to that of a watermelon at birth. The weight of the uterus will increase from 1 ounce now to over 2-1/4 pounds at birth.

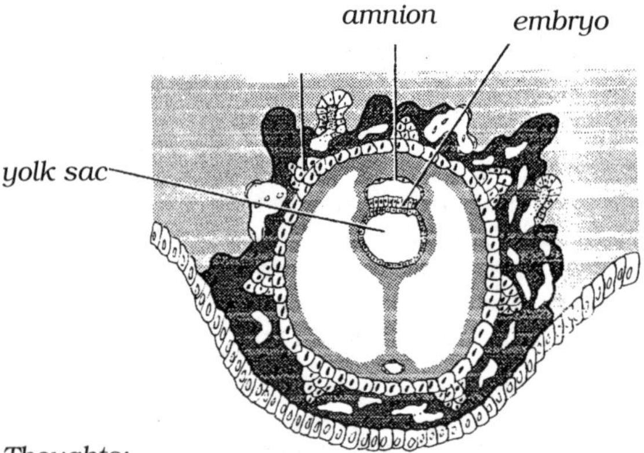

Thoughts:

....

....

DAY 15

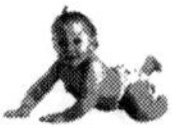

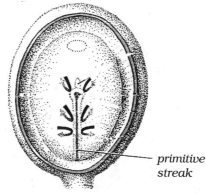

Now the "primitive streak" develops which is the initial parsing of the cells that will become all the organ systems, bones, nerves and skin of the body.

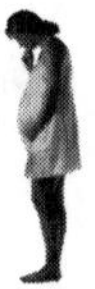

Magnesium is a trace mineral stored in the bones of adults. Magnesium helps build bones and teeth, and regulate insulin and blood sugar levels. 300 mg of magnesium is the recommended daily amount. Magnesium is found in beans, nuts (especially pumpkin seeds), seafoods, and yogurt.

Anatomists from the middle ages thought that babies resulted from uterine growth of miniature men or "homunculi" present in sperm. According to this theory, all the organ systems were already developed in miniature form in sperm.

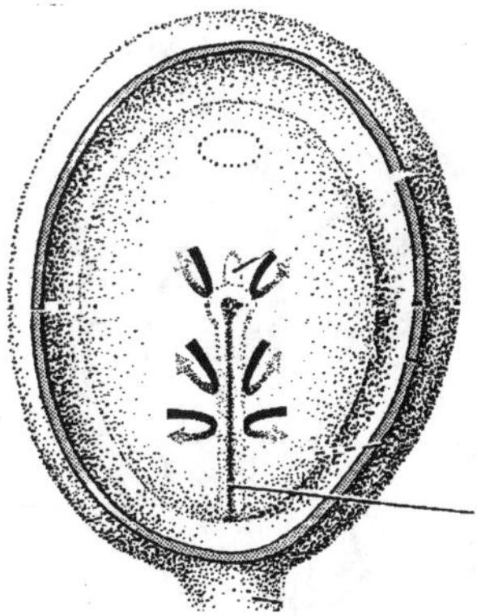

Notes:

....

....

DAY 16

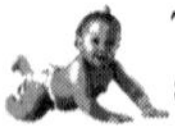

The "primitive knot" develops at the top of the primitive streak. This is the very beginning of the brain and spinal cord. Trained embryologists can now determine the top and bottom, and left and right sides of the embryo.

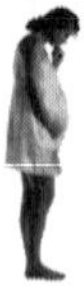

Selection of health care professional - The main sources used to help select prenatal care are personal physician referrals, word of mouth recommendations and referrals from the hospital. When those considerations are made here's what people decide to do for prenatal care and the birth:

80% select an Obstetrician/gynecologist
10% select a general practitioner
5% choose to give birth at home
5% select a Certified Nurse Midwife

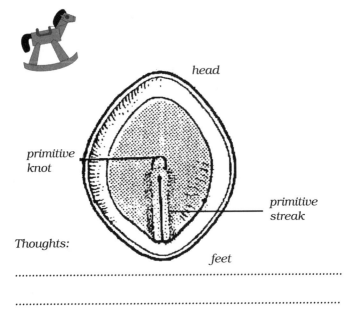

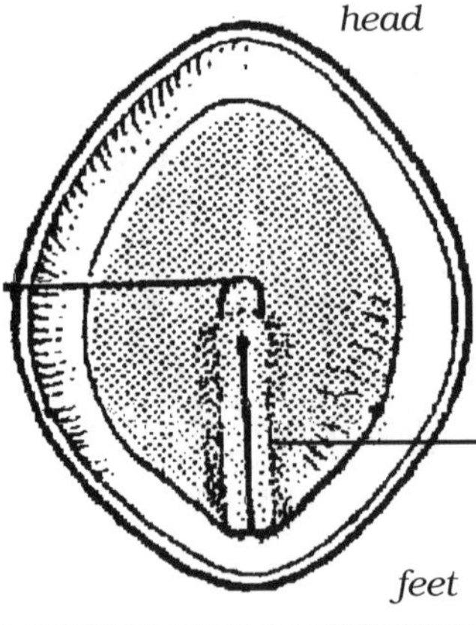

Thoughts:

....

....

DAY 17

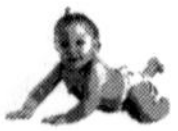

Now there are 3 distinct layers of cells from which all the organ systems and bones develop. These layers are known as the ectoderm, mesoderm and endoderm which mean outer 'skin,' middle 'skin' and inner 'skin.'

Ectoderm: becomes the nervous system (brain and spinal cord), and the skin
Mesoderm: becomes muscles, skeleton, blood, reproductive and excretory organs.
Endoderm: becomes the respiratory system, digestive system, and organs such as liver, stomach, lungs.

cross sectional view through the embryo

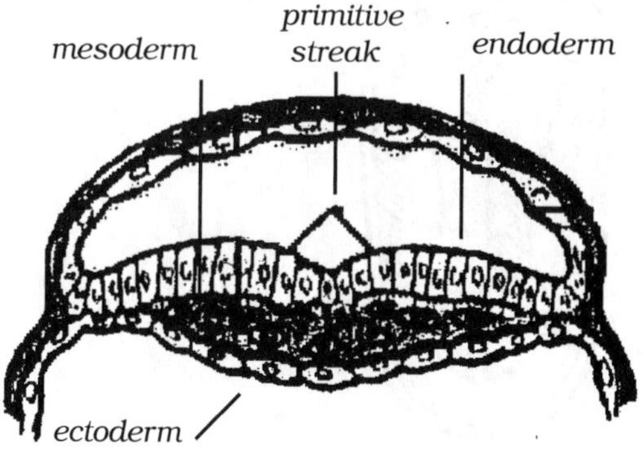

Notes:

....

....

DAY 18

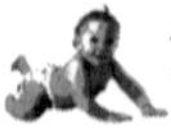

A structure known as the notochord develops that will guide the development of the spinal cord in the baby. As the bones of the spinal column (vertebrae) are formed, the notochord will disappear, having accomplished its goal of providing the "map" for the proper formation of the spinal cord. The notochord also has a role in initiating the formation of the group of cells (the neural plate) that will grow and differentiate into the brain.

The embryo is 1.5 mm in length.

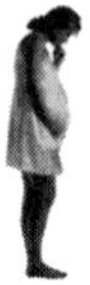

Some women start to experience nausea even at this very early stage. Some find that eating smaller meals more frequently lessens the queasy feelings.

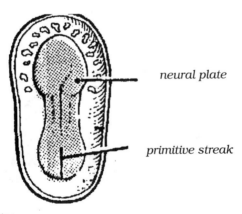

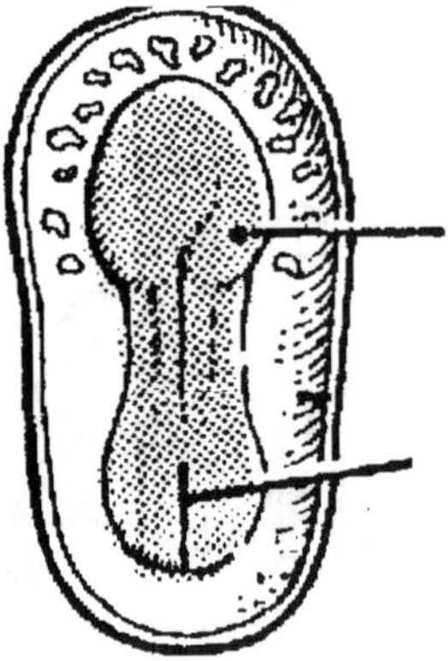

Thoughts:

....

....

DAY 19

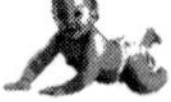

The cardiogenic area, where the heart muscle develops, is located at the top end (head end) of the embryo. Believe it or not, within a day or two the heart will form and start beating, pumping primitive blood throughout the embryo. The precursor of blood (blood cells and plasma) is being formed within the embryo by structures known as blood islands. The liver will start to manufacture blood at about 6 weeks.

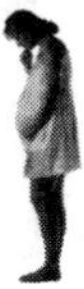

Drinking plenty of liquids may settle your stomach. Plain crackers, toast, or ginger ale may also be soothing.

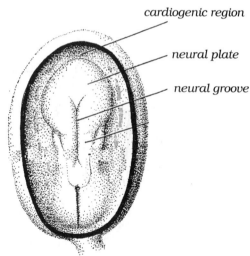

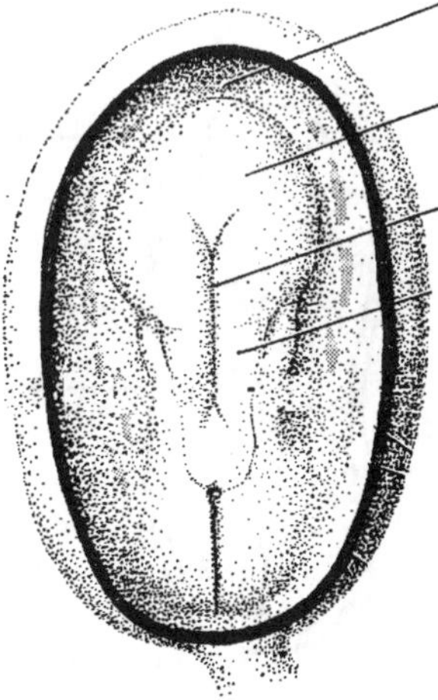

Notes:

....

....

DAY 20

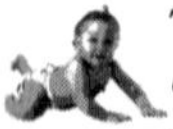

The first somite appears as a small dot in the middle of the embryo. Somites mark the beginning of the development of the skeleton of the head and trunk, the muscles associated with these regions, and the dermis of the skin. Within a week, 42 to 44 pairs of somites will develop. The thyroid gland, which is a chief regulator of cellular activity and metabolism, starts to form.

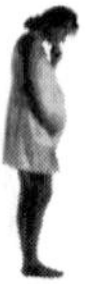

You may feel more tired as your body forces you to slow down and rest.

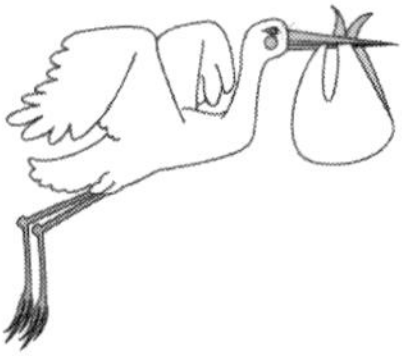

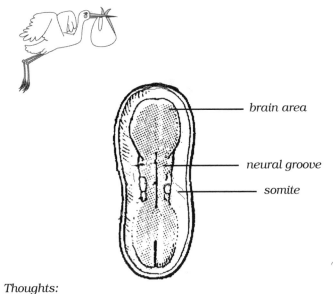

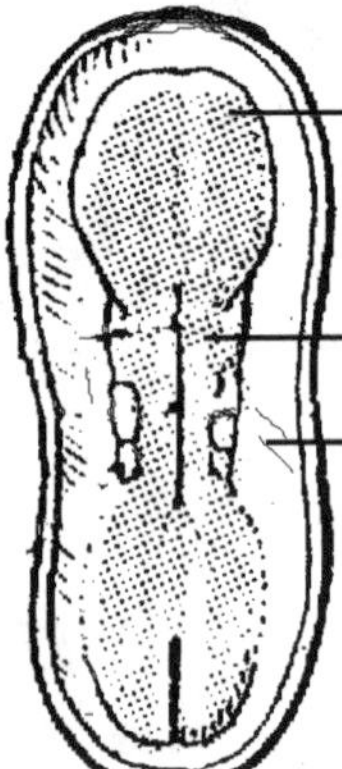

Thoughts:

....

....

DAY 21

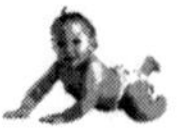

Enough blood has been made to form an early cardiovascular system between the connecting stalk (which becomes the umbilical cord), the chorion, and the vessels and heart of the embryo. The cardiovascular system is the first organ system to reach a functional state - not bad for 3 weeks work!

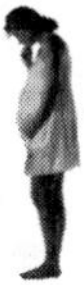

Even at this early stage you may find the need to urinate more. This is due, in part, to more efficient metabolism and the ability to eliminate water products more quickly.

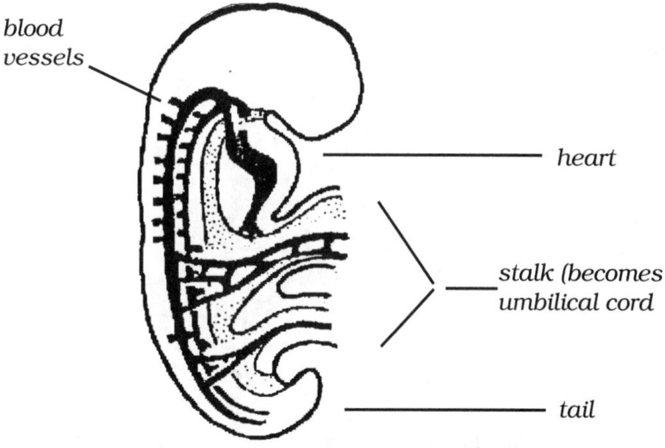

cross section of embryo showing inside

Notes:

....

....

DAY 22

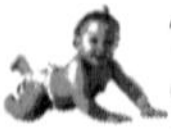

The heart is now beating, pumping early blood through the embryo, cord and yolk sac. Embryonic organ systems, like the heart, form as they function, meaning they operate even as they are developing into a more mature form. The embryo is almost straight in appearance. There is a row of 8 - 10 paired somites now. The liver starts to form now and will occupy most of the abdominal cavity up to Week 10.

Length is .1 inch.

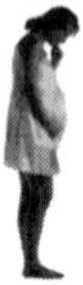

Chromium is a less well-known dietary mineral that is important during pregnancy. Chromium stimulates protein growth in your baby. One slice of whole wheat bread, an apple or some chicken would give you almost a day's supply.

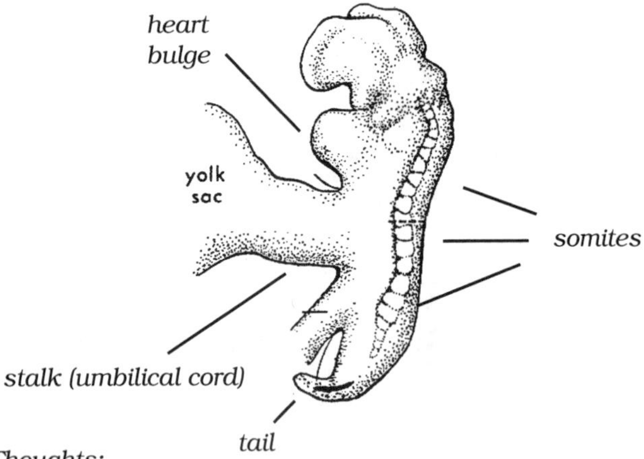

Thoughts:

....

....

DAY 23

The very early beginnings of the eye and ear are present today. The neuropore (early spinal cord) is open at both the top and bottom ends. Soon the embryo will start to take its familiar C-shaped or curled-up appearance, as growth occurs rapidly within the confines of the uterus.

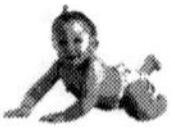

Many women rely on recommendations from family and friends when selecting an obstetrician or obstetrical team. Skill and training is your major concern, but also you'll need to find a doctor or medical team that you're comfortable with.

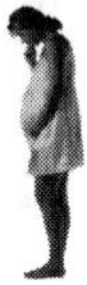

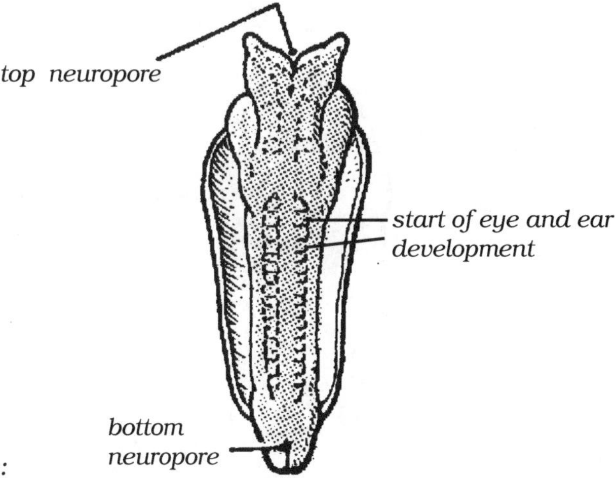

Notes:

....

....

DAY 24

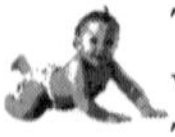

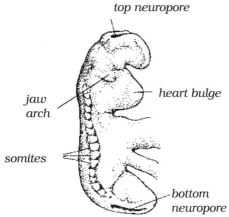

The top neuropore closes as the spinal cord starts to develop. The makings of the jaw are forming in the "jaw arch." The tail is becoming less conspicuous as the embryo lengthens.

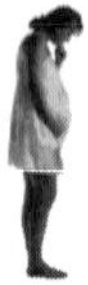

Questions you'll want to ask the doctor include: What are your back-up and on-call arrangements? What services are offered through your office? What prenatal diagnostic tests do you recommend, and why? What are your procedures for labor? What's your thinking about pain medication, epidurals, episiotomies and Caesarians? The answers should be presented in a way that you and your spouse can easily understand. These are important questions because some of these tests and procedures may be performed on you or the baby.

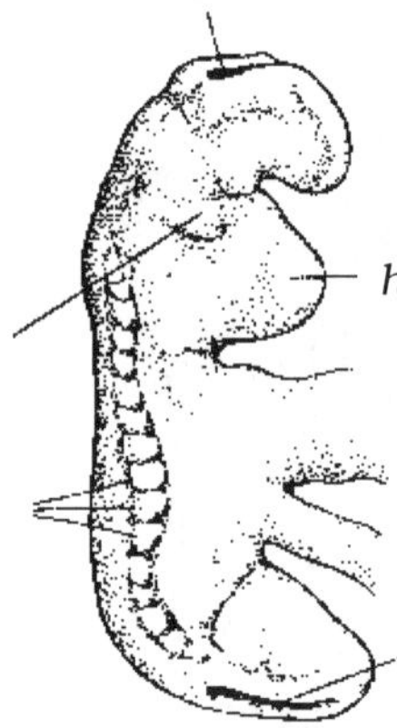

Thoughts:

Remember to use this area to jot down questions

to ask your healthcare provider at your appointments

DAY 25

There are now about 20 somites visible on the embryo, making way for the development of bones, skin and organs. The chorionic villi are well-developed, enabling vascular communication between mother and embryo.

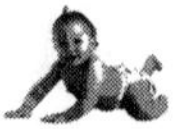

About half of all pregnant women experience morning sickness between Weeks 5 - 15. The range of symptoms can be from a mild queasy feeling to incapacitating vomiting. If you experience severe morning sickness, it is important that you make your doctor aware of this. Good nutrition is essential for your growing baby. Your doctor, nurse or midwife can help you reduce the feelings of nausea.

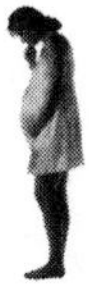

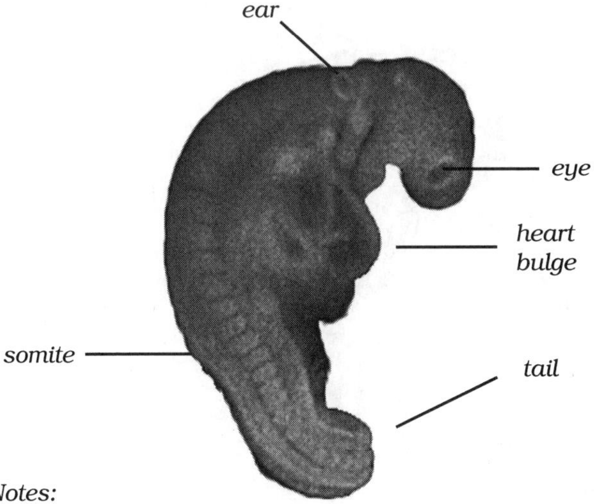

Notes:

....

....

DAY 26

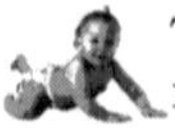

The main divisions of the central nervous system are present now. The spinal cord, hindbrain, midbrain and forebrain are developing. The beginnings of the arms appear in the form of arm buds. The eye and ear canal are clearly visible. The bottom neuropore is closed. The tongue forms, and the beginnings of the lung - the lung bud - appears now.

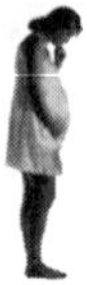

Causes of morning sickness : A combination of changes in your body to support the pregnancy are probably to blame. Increased estrogen, progesterone, enhanced sense of smell and taste, and increased fatigue can all contribute.

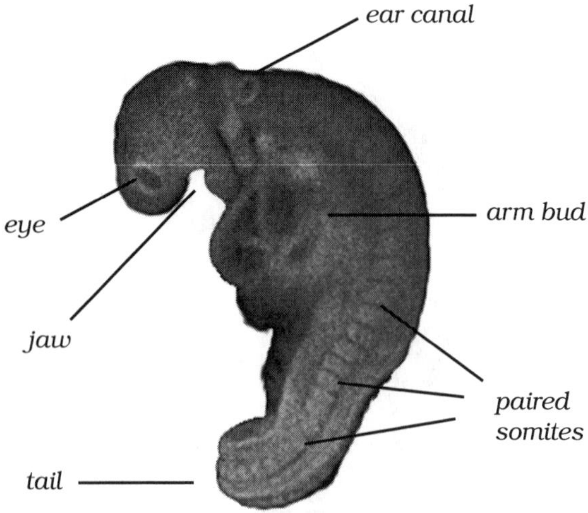

Thoughts:

....

....

DAY 27

Now the prominence of the forebrain is noticeable as well as a clear and distinct arm bud. From this side view you can also see the tail, the ear and eye.

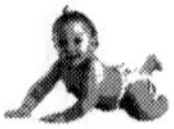

Your baby's brain and nervous system will undergo rapid growth in the next few weeks. Folic acid, one of the B vitamins, has been shown to be very important in normal neural development. Green leafy vegetables and fortified breads and cereals are excellent sources of folic acid.

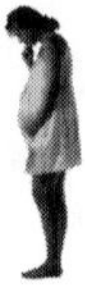

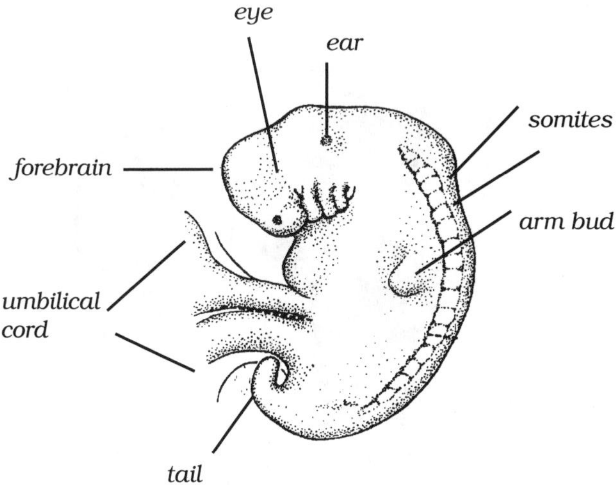

Notes:

....

....

DAY 28

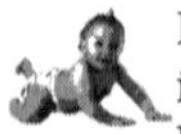

From this front-on view the embryo is starting to look familiar. You can see a true head, eyes, and chest area. The heart has its ventricles and atria. The tail is still prominent, and will eventually become the coccyx of the spinal column. Today starts the beginning of the process that will produce a recognizable face. Folds of tissue in the head region will bend and fuse. The seams of these fusions make the mouth, ear holes, the flair of the nostrils and the little ridge between the nose and upper lip (the philstrum).

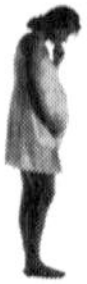

Morning sickness can occur morning, noon and night. Most women experience a marked decline in nausea by the end of the third month but specific odors can trigger a bout of nausea any time if you're queasy.

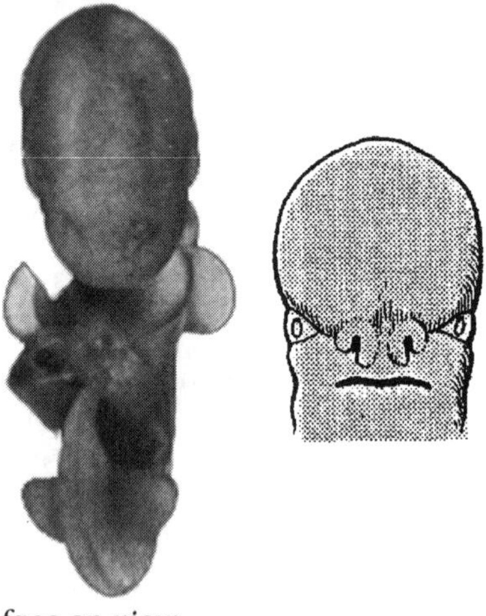

Thoughts: *face-on view*

....

....

DAY 29

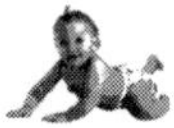

Today the legs start to form as leg buds, just like the arms did earlier. The arms are lengthening. The lens of the eye, which will focus light on the light-receptive part of the eye, the retina, is forming. The tail is starting to become much smaller and will disappear soon. As a reference, the embryo is about the size of an apple seed.

Length is 1/2 inch .10 oz.

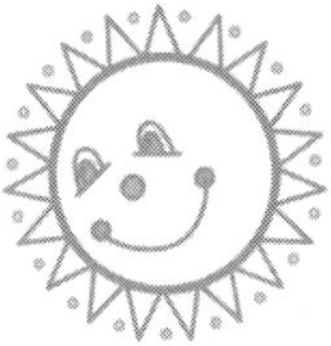

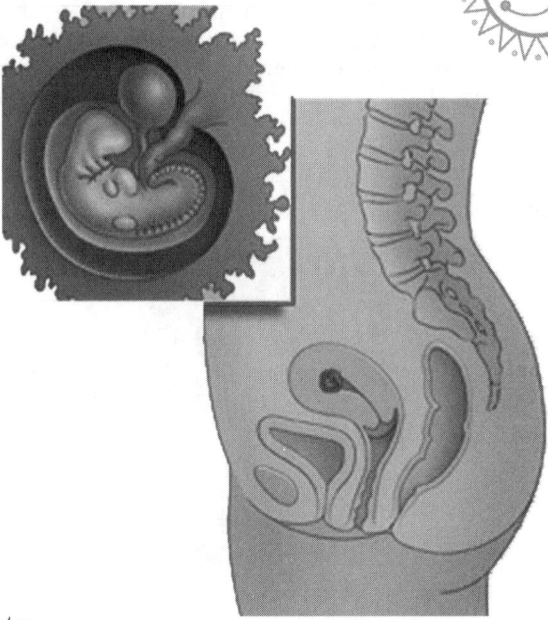

Notes:

....

....

DAY 30

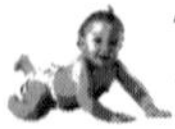

The ear parts that you can see will become the inner ears as the embryo develops. The eyes are actually on the sides of the head and will move forward to the front of the face as the baby develops. The diaphragm - the drum-like sheet of elastic tissue involved in breathing - develops these next few days.

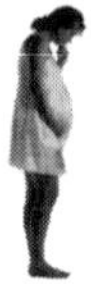

First prenatal visit - A complete medical history will be taken and you'll be given a physical exam. Heart rate, blood pressure and blood tests will screen for problems and establish baselines for reference throughout your pregnancy. Another pregnancy test will also be ordered just to make sure that you're pregnant.

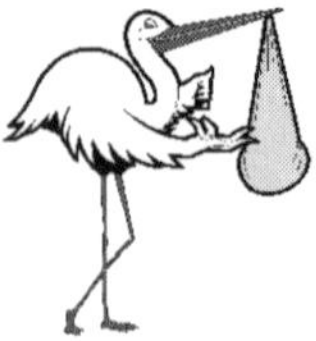

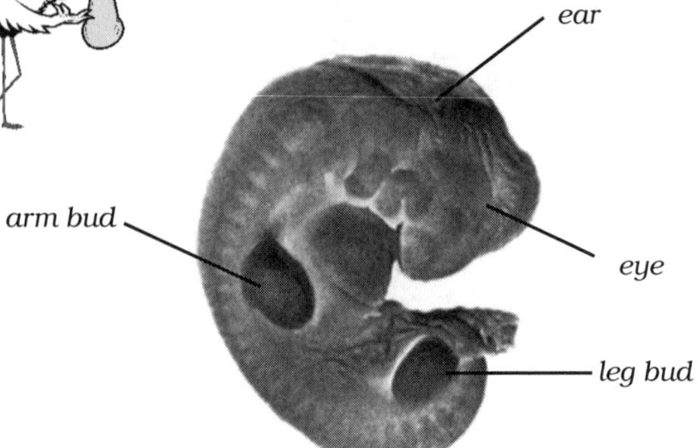

Thoughts:

....

....

DAY 31

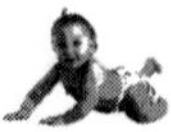

Now there are about 30 pairs of somites running almost the entire length of the embryo. The yolk sac is still connected to the embryo but will soon be replaced by the umbilical cord. The cord will have two umbilical arteries and one umbilical vein. The path of the umbilical vein is still present in the adult as a string of tissue stretching from the navel to the liver. The bottom image is an ultrasound rendering of the implanted embryo.

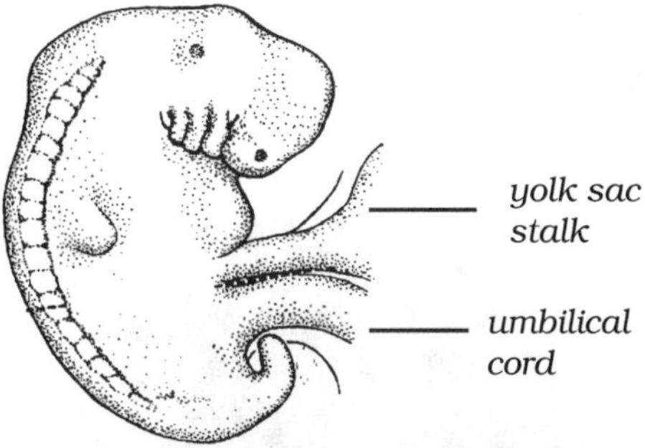

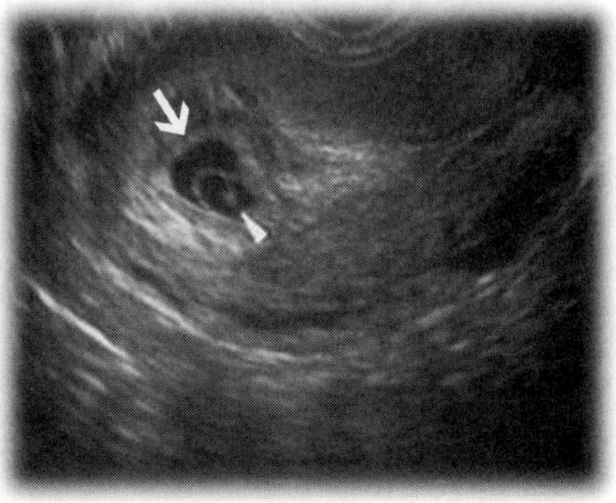

DAY 32

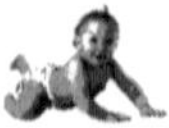

Notice that the arm bud is developing a rounded end - this is the beginning of the hand taking shape. Also the mouth opening starts to form.

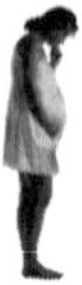

Your skin will change during the course of the pregnancy. Increased production and secretion of oil will make your skin more pliable for stretching. Most women experience an improvement in their complexion during pregnancy.

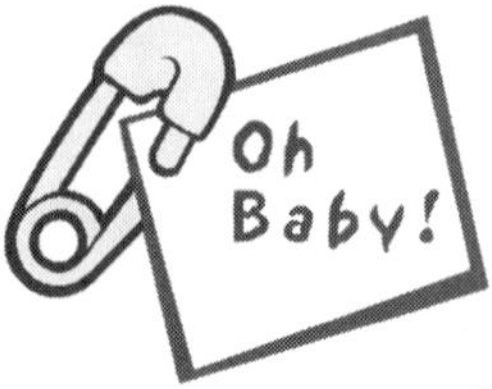

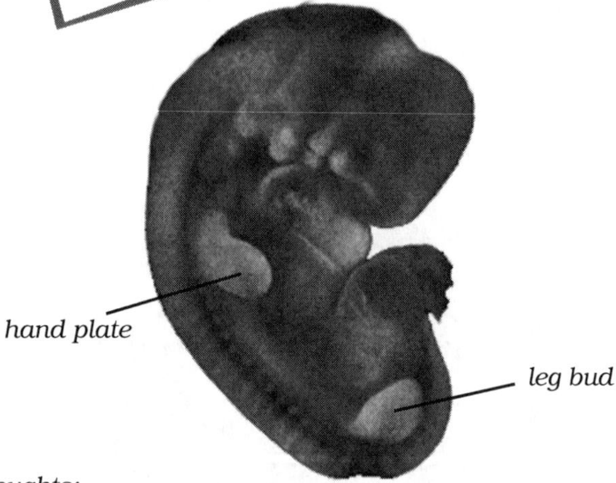

Thoughts:

....

....

DAY 33

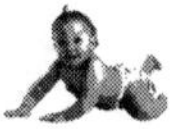

The maximum number of somites are now present, ranging from 35-48 pairs. The mouth area and jaw is clearly visible, with the outer angles of the mouth clearly defined. The embryo is 1/2 inch long, curved along the length of its characteristic C-shape.

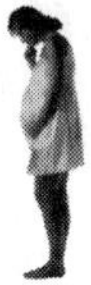

A type of bacteria (helicobacter pylori) that causes stomach ulcers may also cause a severe form of morning sickness. Over 90% of women with a severe form of morning sickness were infected with the bacteria. Some scientists think that during the early phases of pregnancy changes in body fluid concentration affect the acidity of the stomach, which may activate dormant bacteria in the stomach.

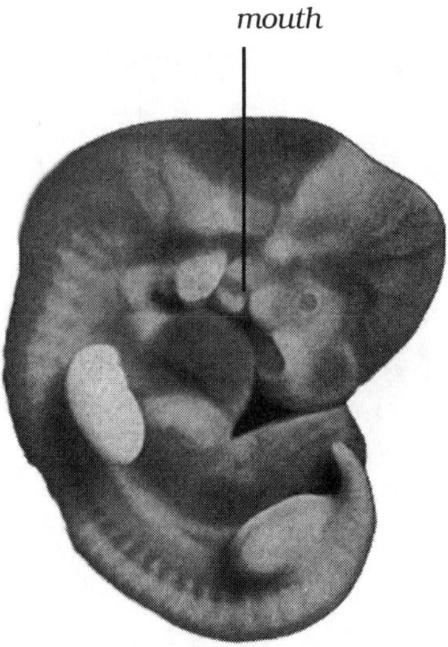

Notes:

....

....

DAY 34

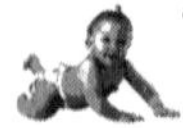

The head is becoming proportionately much larger compared to the trunk. The eye is developing some detail with the lens forming as well as some of the pigmented (colored) iris. The heart has developed its characteristic two-sided form with arterial output and venous return.

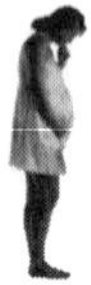

Many women experience some change in their cognitive capabilities during the course of a pregnancy. Most common is increased forgetting. Earlier it was chalked up to distraction, as it would be expected a mother would think/daydream about her new baby. New research has found that a woman's brain actually shrinks 3-5% during pregnancy. Most of the shrinkage is due to water loss. But don't worry, your brain returns to its normal size about 6 months after birth.

The word 'embryo' comes from the Greek 'to grow, to swell.'

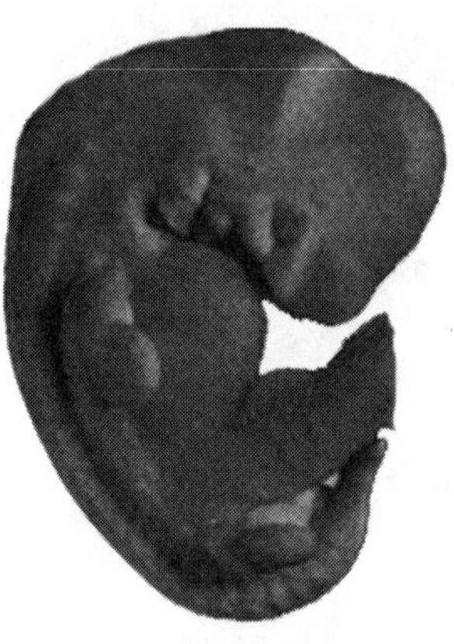

Thoughts:

....

....

DAY 35

The leg bud has developed a foot plate that will form the foot and toes. A face-on view shows that the nostrils are formed but positioned wider than their final location. The liver is now forming blood in blood islands.

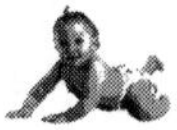

What could be the 'adaptive value' of morning sickness? Some think that the nausea may promote energy storage by decreasing activity (but then why throw up?) Others think the nausea may lead to a more varied diet - you are less likely to eat something again if you 'think' it may have made you sick. One final thought: If the nausea had survival value, chances are all women would experience it; they don't.

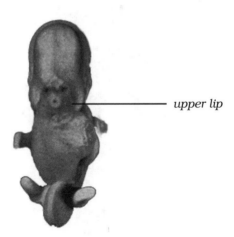

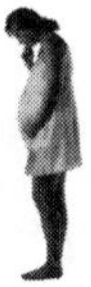

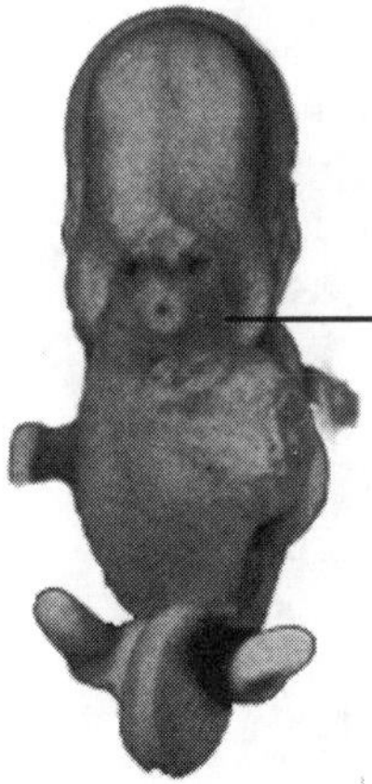

Notes:

....

....

DAY 36

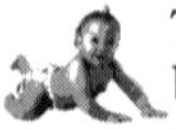

This view from behind shows that the arm has developed a bend in it today - the elbow has formed. Some of the first movements - arching the back and neck - are seen now. As a reference, the embryo is now about the size of a blueberry.

Baby is 3/4 inch ❦ .15 oz.

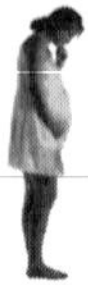

Pyridoxine, or Vitamin B_6 ,relieves morning sickness for some women. B_6 helps the body metabolize amino acids (proteins). 25 mg taken in the morning, mid-afternoon and at bedtime reduced symptoms for women experiencing severe nausea. Good dietary sources of B_6 are meats, poultry, fish, potatoes and whole grains. How B_6 works to decrease nausea is unknown.

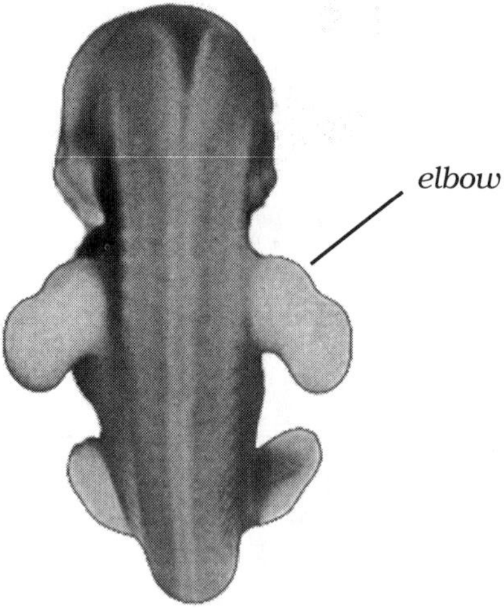

Thoughts:

....

....

DAY 37

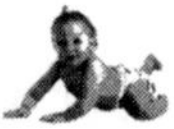

Today the hand plate is 'pinching-in' to form the fingers - webbed fingers. The head will also increase in size due to the rapid brain growth. This pushes the head down against the heart. The skeleton is forming, first as a continuous joint-less cartilagineous model. Later bone will form, as specialized cells extract calcium from the blood to cast the bone.

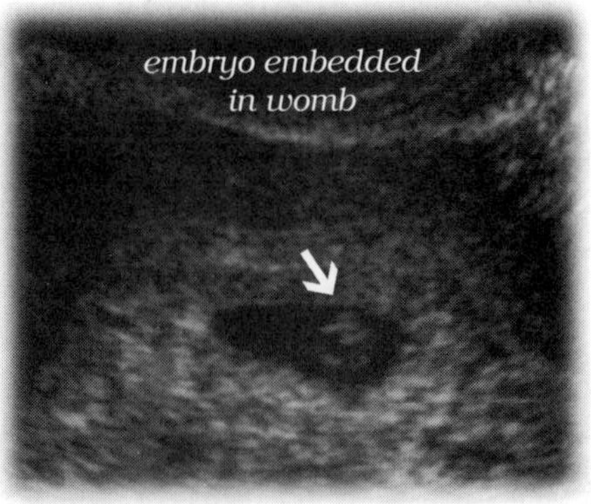

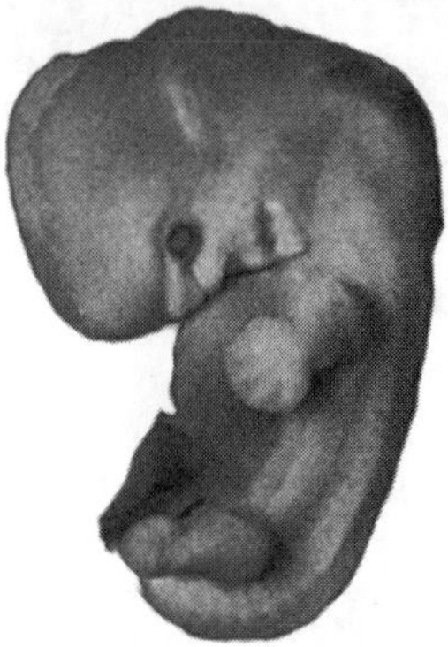

DAY 38

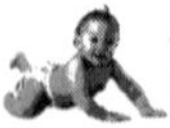

A touch to the mouth area causes the head to turn away in the other direction. This is the first demonstration of an avoidance or protective reflex. The upper lip is formed showing a clear separation from the nostrils. The tip of the nose is seen in profile. Nostrils are widely separated and will start to move together now. The hand is taking shape with the appearance of finger buds. The foot is paddle-shaped.

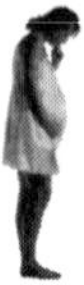

In Europe, 75% of births are attended by midwives. In the US, only 5%. While you're pregnant you won't ovulate because the hormonal environment has changed now that you're pregnant. Your body knows it's pregnant so why bother. Other biochemical changes may occur that could make you feel more irritable or even depressed, even though you are excited about having a baby.

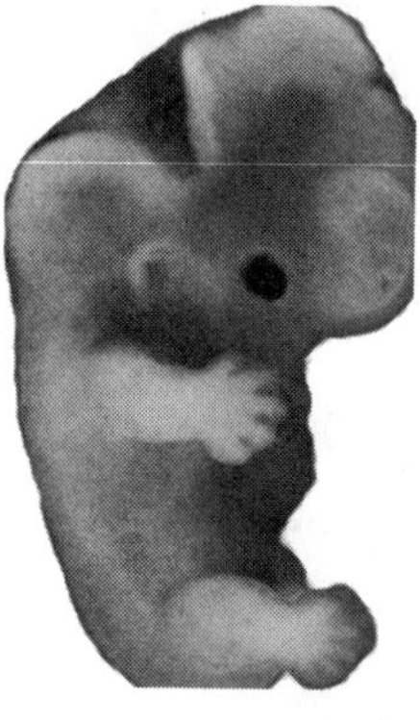

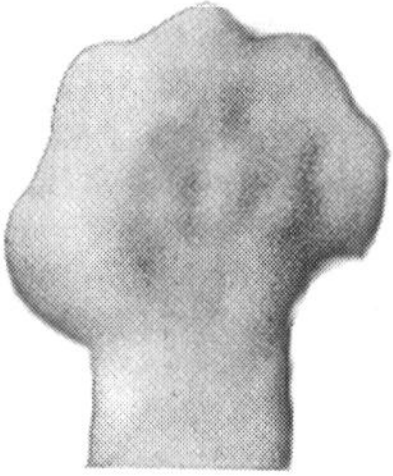

Hand

Thoughts:

....

....

DAY 39

Pigmentation or color appears in the eyes for the first time. The outer ear, the pinna, is present under 'the chin.' It will migrate to its position on the side of the head over the next week or so. Cerebrospinal fluid (which flows through the open spaces of the brain) forms now.

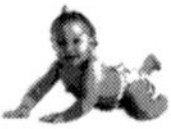

Potassium, an essential mineral, is important in neural transmission and fluid balance. Bananas are an excellent source of potassium as is watermelon, baked potatoes, raisins and mushrooms.

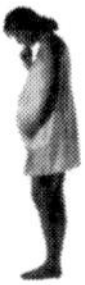

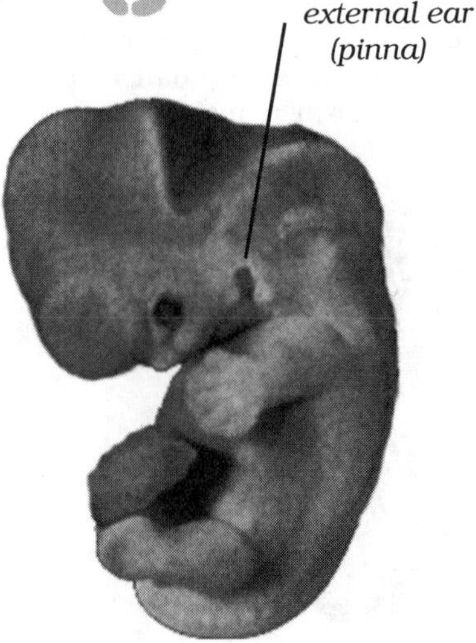

Notes:

....

....

DAY 40

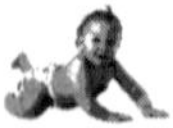

"A person's a person, no matter how small." -
Dr. Seuss, Horton Hears a Who.

The first detectable brain waves are recordable today. This means that brain function is working in a complex coordinated manner with neurons activated in organized and functional patterns. Can the embryo think? Is there consciousness? No one knows for sure. The palate, the roof of the mouth, is developing today. The facial muscles are starting to form - soon the baby will be making facial expressions. The fingers are almost separated.

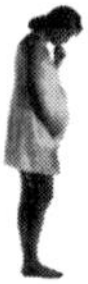

Some women feel their nausea subside when they miss taking their maternity vitamins. For some women these vitamins could be causing nausea. Only your doctor can assess the risks vs. the benefits of taking your vitamin supplement if you feel the vitamin makes you nauseous. Eating a well-balanced diet is a good way to make sure your baby gets the nutrients it needs.

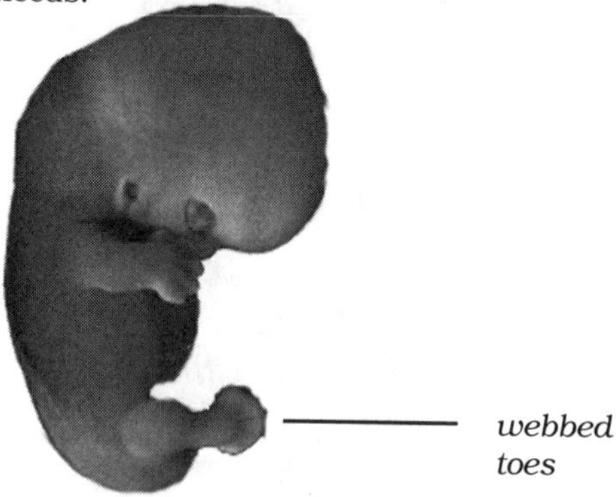

Thoughts:

....

....

DAY 41

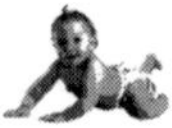

From this face-on view you can see the tips of the fingers and the placement of the eyes slightly on the sides of the head. The liver is now forming blood that will enter into the general circulation. Nerve fibers from the cerebral cortex form into a band (the internal capsule) and descend to the spinal cord. These neural cables will enable voluntary movement.

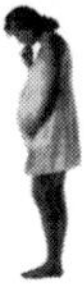

Your blood volume will increase almost 50% over the next month and a half. You may notice veins becoming more pronounced in your legs, breasts and torso as your skin stretches.

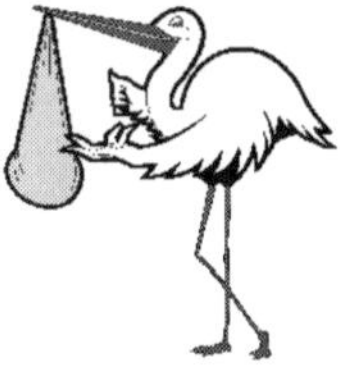

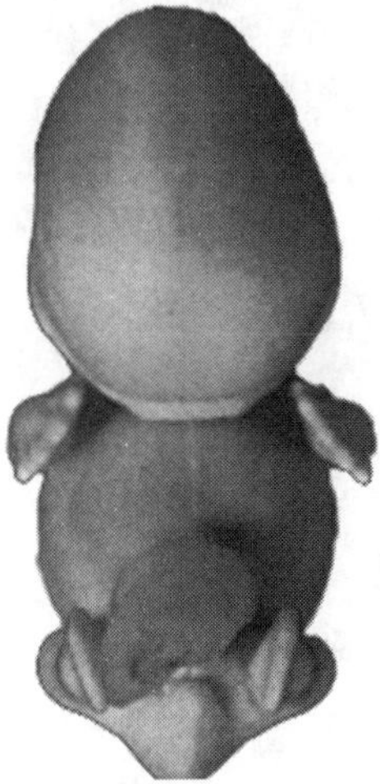

Notes:

....

....

DAY 42

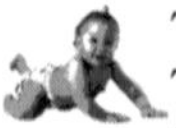

The toes are now distinctly formed but they are still webbed. The posture is also changing as the leg area straightens out. Soon the C-shape of the baby will be lost. The pancreas forms now and will secrete insulin in 2 weeks.

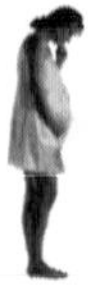

Almost all women (90%) develop stretch marks during their pregnancy. Gradual weight gain and keeping your skin moisturized will diminish the impact and occurrence of stretch marks.

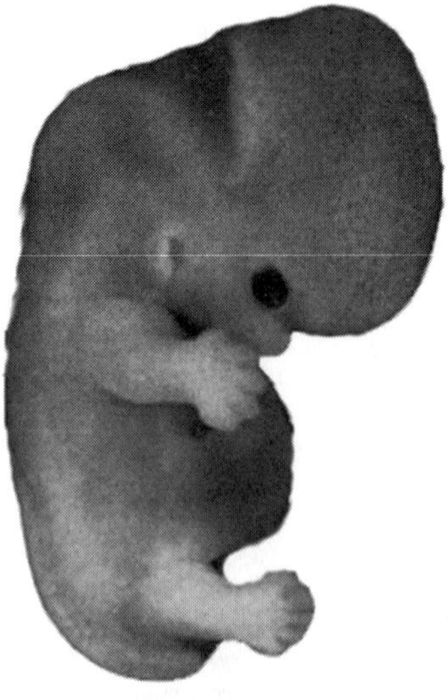

Thoughts:

....

....

DAY 43

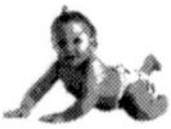

Eyelids are starting to form around the ridges of the eyes. The trunk is elongating and straightening. The thyroid gland in the neck now secretes calcitonin to regulate calcium levels in the body. The main thyroid hormone, thyroxin, won't develop until Week 18. As a reference, the embryo is now about the size of a raspberry.

Baby is 1 inch ❦ 1/4 oz.

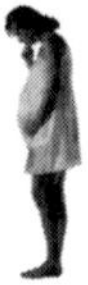

Pregnancy requires that you take in more iron each day, about 18 mg total. Red meat, eggs, green vegetables and whole wheat breads contain iron. Dried raisins, apricots and peaches contain substantial iron. Iron can cause constipation, so eat more fiber and drink more water if you're taking iron supplements.

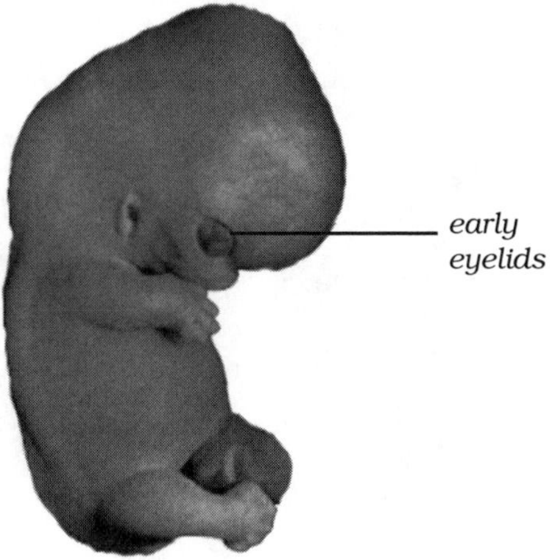

Notes:

....

....

DAY 44

The tip of the nose is distinct. The cartilage that has given structure to the embryo is now starting to turn into bone. The first regions to ossify or harden are the shoulder blades (clavicle) then the jaw and palate are next. A sex difference is present as females show ossification sooner than male babies. The pinna or external ear is taking shape. The hand has distinctly separate fingers and fingertips.

Legumes such as peas, beans and lentils contain protein, iron, thiamin (B_1) and riboflavin (B_2). Legumes are a great all around nutritional source. Riboflavin is essential for your baby's muscle, bone and nerve development.

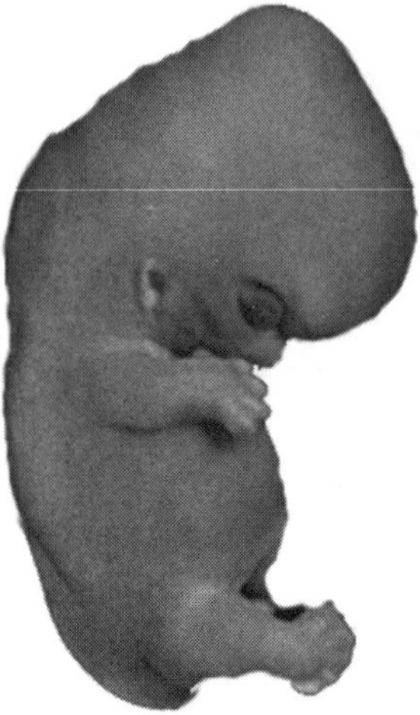

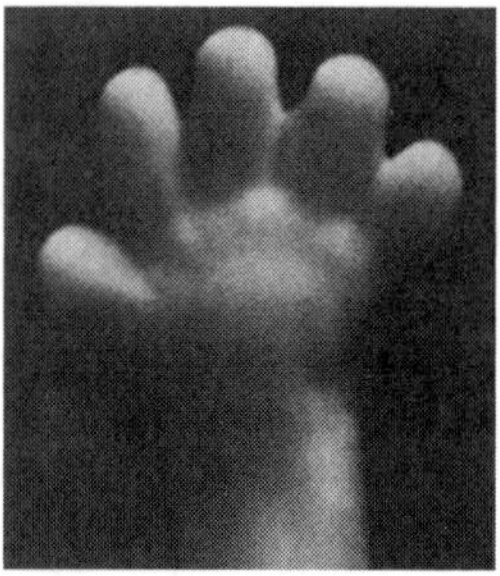

Thoughts:

....

....

DAY 45

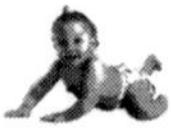

The arm is bent at the elbow. Nipples are formed on both males and females. Lots of self-generated, spontaneous movements like twitching and shaking (initiated within the spinal cord) are present. Both limbs move together, with the signal to contract the muscles coming from the spinal cord. In a few weeks, the control of movement will transfer to the brain.

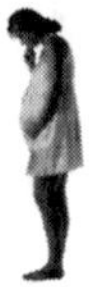

Many women have a 'mental image' of their baby by now. Some studies have shown that women who bond with their babies prenatally are more happy and competent caregivers after the birth.

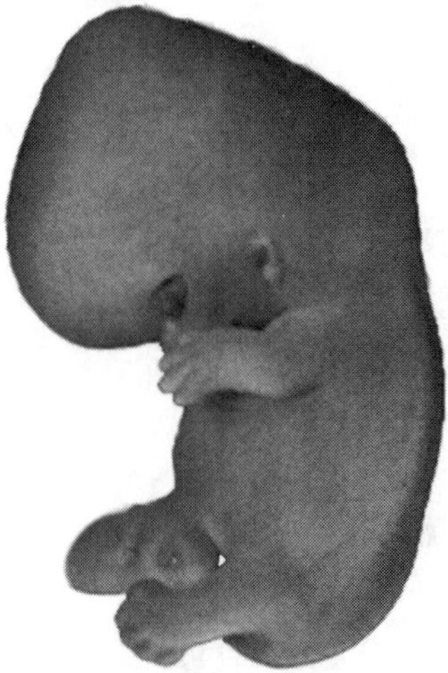

Notes:

....

....

DAY 46

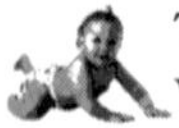

The gonads (ovaries or testes) are starting to develop deep within the abdominal cavity. The testes will migrate out into the scrotum later. As the connections between the fast growing brain, nerves and muscles continue, the baby will start to make small voluntary movements...just testing out the wiring to make sure it works.

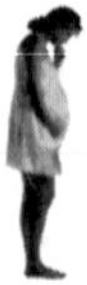

Water retention and swelling (edema), most noticeably in the feet and ankles, is a normal part of pregnancy. Your baby's increasing weight, plus your extra blood volume, combine to create pressure that slows down circulation. When you sit or stand in one place for too long gravity compounds the situation. Don't wear tight, restrictive clothing. Taking a rest with your feet elevated may reduce the swelling.

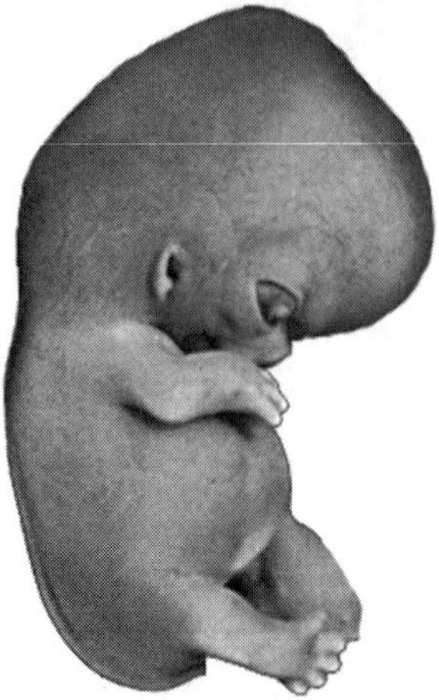

Thoughts:

....

....

DAY 47

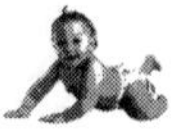

The brain is growing at the rate of 100,000 new neurons per minute. The skin over the wrists, knees and ankles puckers where the folding and development of these joints is occurring. The esophagus and trachea develop now.

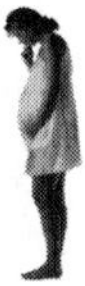

Nasal congestion is common during pregnancy as the mucous membranes become more vascularized and swell. This is due, in part, to the greater levels of estrogen in your body now. You may also be more prone to nosebleeds as well.

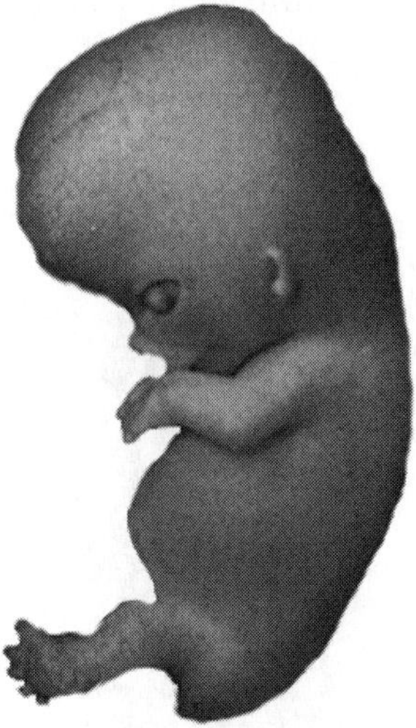

Notes:

....

....

DAY 48

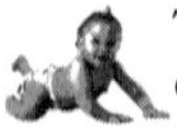

The fingers are almost completely separated (webs of skin exist about half-way up the fingers). The fingers have touch pads - enlarged surfaces on the finger tips that will regress. The nasal cavity is a separate chamber from the mouth. Specialized cells called chemoreceptors are present in the nasal cavity. These cells detect substances suspended in the amniotic fluid now, and airborne molecules after birth.

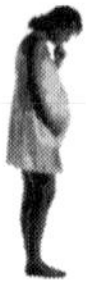

New aches and pains are a normal accompaniment to pregnancy. In addition to compensating for the additional weight you're carrying, you may also feel twinges as the ligaments supporting your uterus stretch. A sudden twinge of pain around the groin area is most likely a fallopian tube spasm. These are normal and will subside in a few weeks.

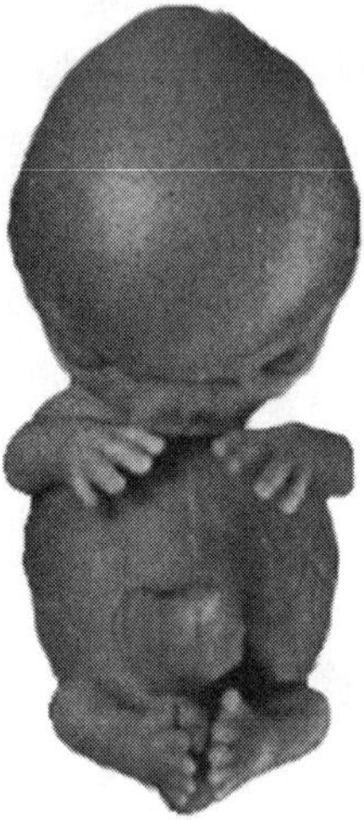

Thoughts:

....

....

DAY 49

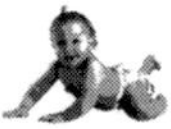

The heart is beating at about 140 - 150 beats per minute, about twice as fast as the mother's heart beat. The legs are lengthening. The tail is almost gone. Touching the skin around the cheek will cause the head to turn away. This is one of the first indications that the brain is functioning to receive outside sensory input (the touch) and initiate appropriate reflexive behavior (the head turn). The baby is responsive to external sensory input and responds with an appropriate behavioral response - not bad for someone only 1-1/2 inches long!

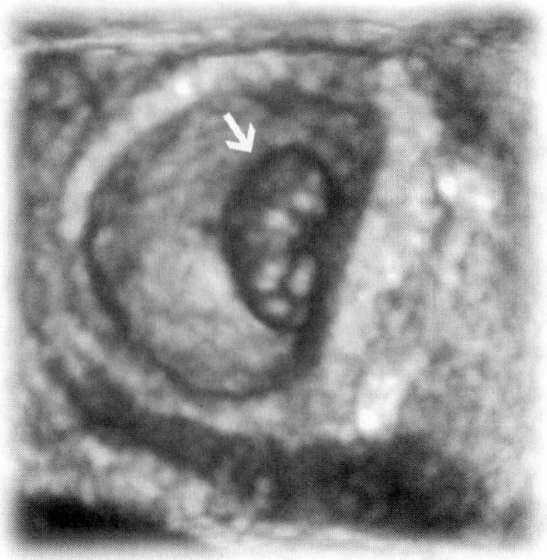

7 week old embryo implanted in uterus

Notes:

....

....

DAY 50

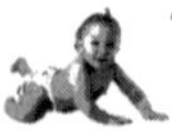

Touching the side of the face causes the mouth to open and the head to turn toward the touch. This is the first approach response. It may be an early component of the rooting reflex that babies show when searching for a nipple. The face is taking on a more human appearance with the elongation of the nose and eyes moving to the front of the head. Fingers have distinct pads and are getting longer and the toes are distinct but webbed. As a point of reference, the baby is now about the same size as a grape.

Baby is 1-1/2 inches ❦ 1/4 oz.

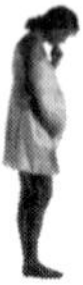

Keep active but don't overdo it when pregnant. Stretching and toning type workouts are best; avoid strenuous workouts. Listen to your body and rest when you're tired.

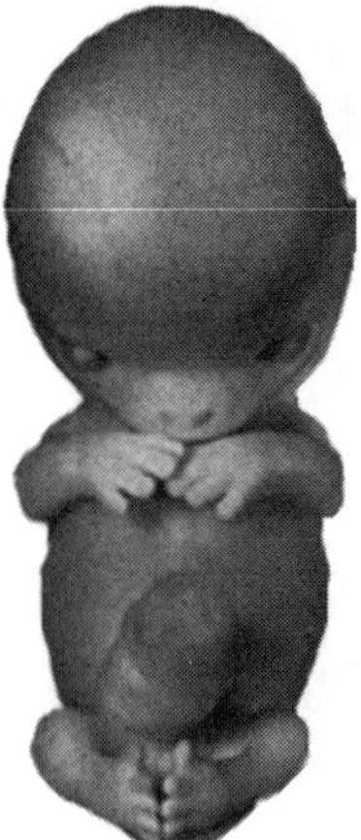

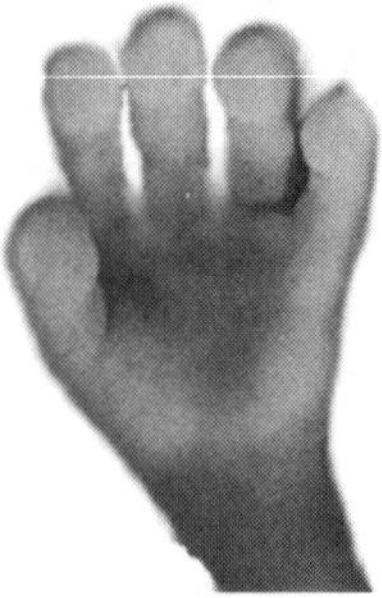

Thoughts:

....

....

DAY 51

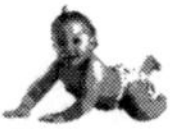

Touching the baby's palm will cause the fingers to bend as shown in B below. The fingers bend at just one joint and the thumb is not involved at all. This is the very beginning of the grasp reflex. Swallowing reflexes involving the tongue are present now. The baby is swallowing amniotic fluid. The swallowing of amniotic fluid shows us the functioning of another system: the baby urinates. This demonstrates that the gastrointestinal tract is functional, as are the kidneys.

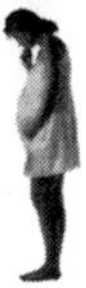

You may have noticed that your nails are growing fast and strong. The improved circulation and metabolism that accompanies pregnancy facilitates nail growth.

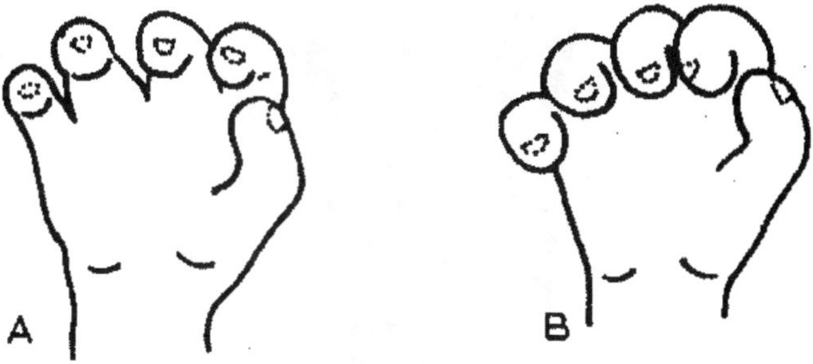

A. Hand at rest

B. Position of the fingers after touching the palm
from Humphrey (1964).

Notes:

....

....

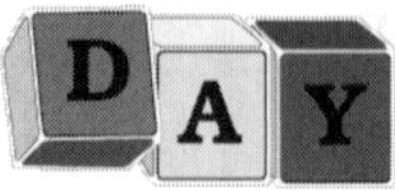

52

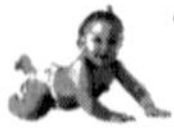

The outer ear or pinna is clearly raised against the side of the head. Both ears develop at exactly the same rate and form the same unique, individualized swirl pattern, all controlled by the genes. The forehead is prominent during this period. Over the next month, the chin and jaw will grow into prominence. The embryo now looks unmistakably human.

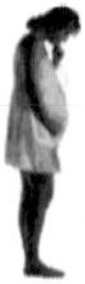

Change your position frequently for optimal circulation. Remaining in one position too long can allow blood to pool. When you rest on your left side, blood flow to the baby and placenta is optimized.

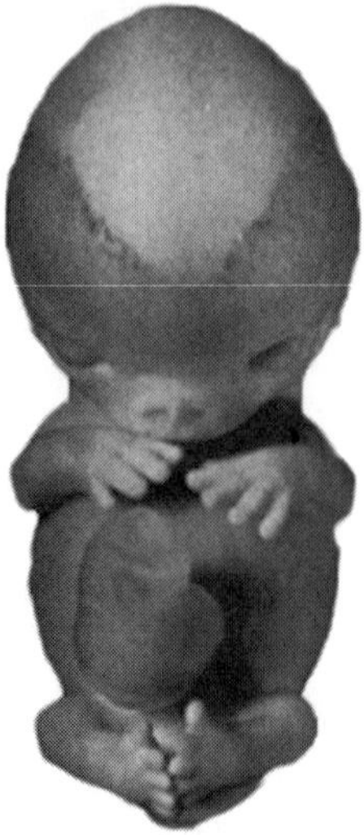

Thoughts:

....

....

DAY 53

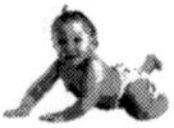

Differentiation of the genitals starts from a common genital tubercle in boys and girls. All the internal organs are present and starting to grow. During this week your baby can move each limb separately: both limbs moved together last week. The bend of the knee is clearly evident and the soles of the feet face each other. A clearly visible change occurs on the scalp with the appearance of the scalp vascular plexus - a seam separating skull bones that can be seen through the skin. The arms are getting longer and bend at the elbows. Lacrimal glands, which will produce tears, form now.

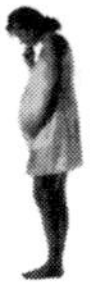

Small, frequent meals will help you maintain a constant energy level without making you feel stuffed and bloated.

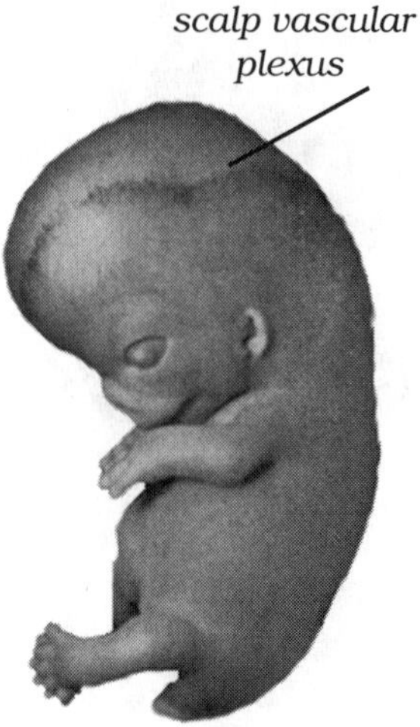

Notes:

....

....

DAY 54

The V-shape on the head is the "soft-spot" on a baby's head (the fontanels). Inside the brain, the cranial nerves are taking shape, with the optic (vision), olfactory bulbs (smell), trigeminal (facial control) regions forming. The stomach has formed and gastric glands that will aid digestion are now developing.

The ultrasound image to the right is similar to what you may see during your first ultrasound examination. The dotted elliptical border is a computer-generated image that will measure the length of the baby. Often the Crown-Rump length is taken because the legs are flexed up toward the abdomen.

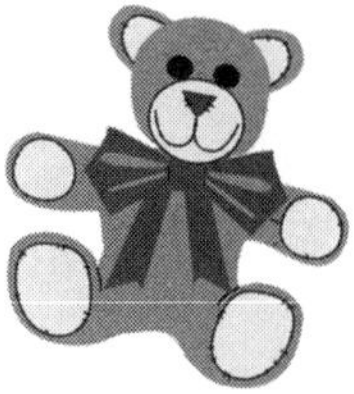

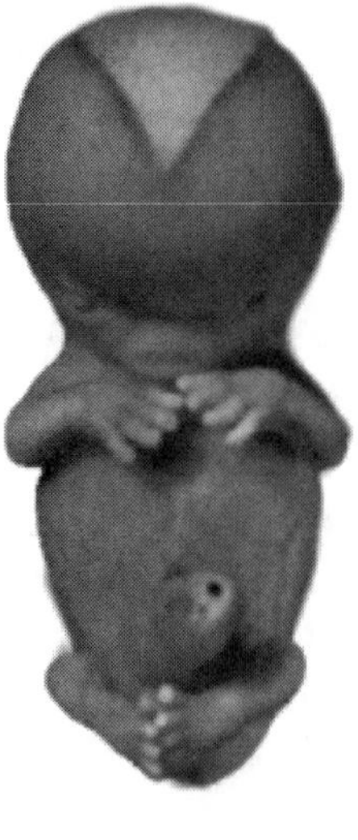

Thoughts:

....

....

DAY 55

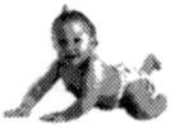

The eyelids are formed and fused together over the eye. The eyes will remain closed until the sixth month. The spinal cord, and all of its associated nerves, are present in miniature form. The arms are long enough that the hands meet in the midline. Fingerprints develop.

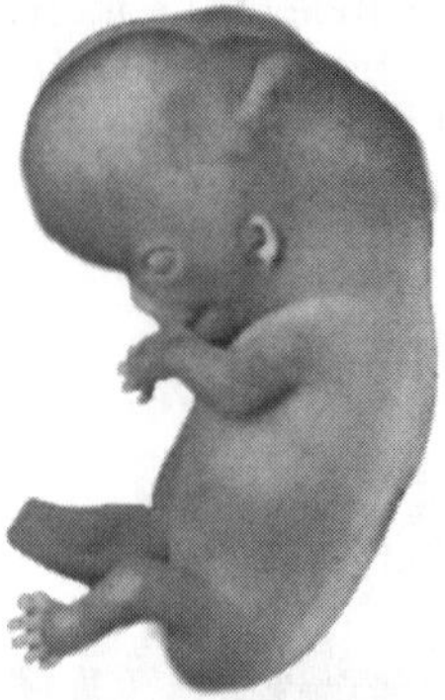

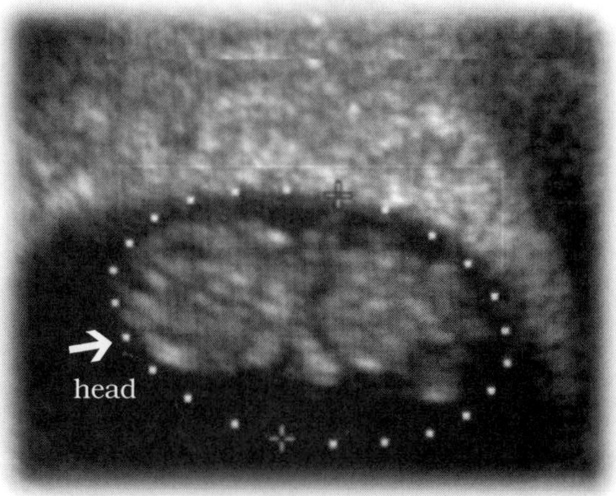

Ultrasound image (embryo facing out)

DAY 56

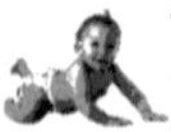

Today the big event is the complete disappearance of the tail. The embryo is now a complete miniature human being that will develop in complexity and size over the next 6 months. The baby now has a distinct neck.

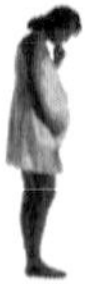

Over the course of the pregnancy your heart rate may increase somewhat because of the increasing cardiovascular demands from the baby. Your health care practitioner will measure your heart rate and blood pressure at each prenatal visit.

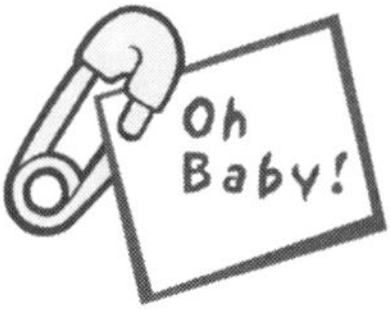

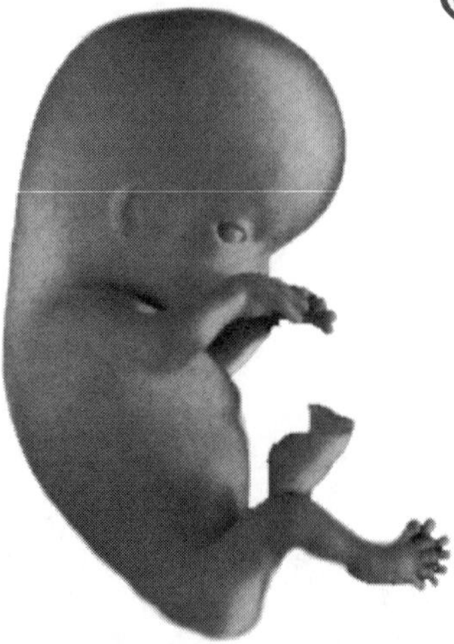

Thoughts:

....

....

DAY 57

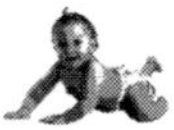

Congratulations! Your embryo is now a fetus and will remain so until birth. Now begins the second trimester of your pregnancy. Fetus means offspring in Greek. As a reference, the baby is about the same size as a strawberry.

Baby is 2 inches ❦ 1/3 oz.

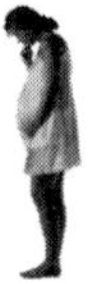

This month's prenatal visit will involve getting your weight and blood pressure measured, general exam and a urine sample for blood sugar levels and proteins. Be sure to bring your list of questions.

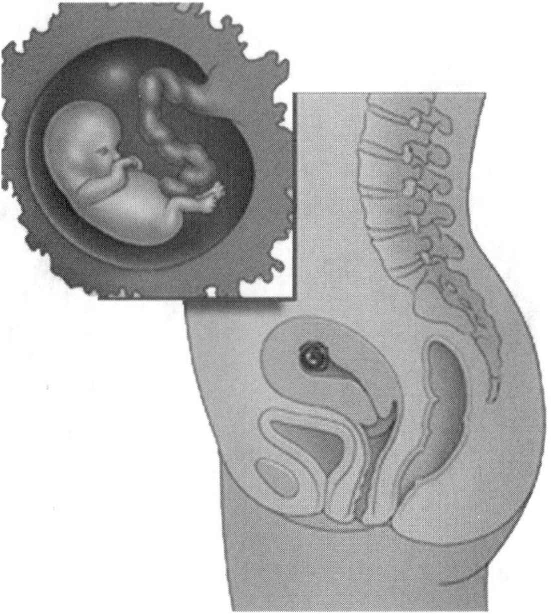

Notes:

....

....

DAY 58

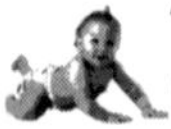

The eyelids have moved closer together and the nose is recognizable from the profile. Notice the distinct bend of the elbow and the almost complete disappearance of the scalp vascular plexus. The toes are separating as the skin constituting the webbing selectively dies away. There is the beginning of an arch on the bottom of the foot and you can see the curvature of the heel. The pituitary gland - also called the master gland - assumes its position in the base of the brain.

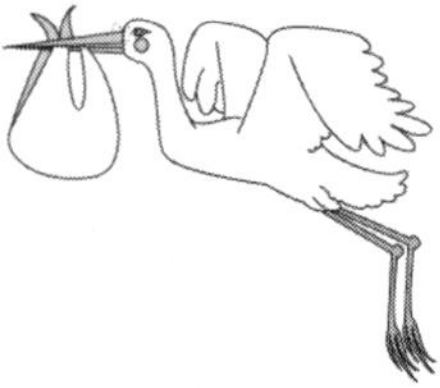

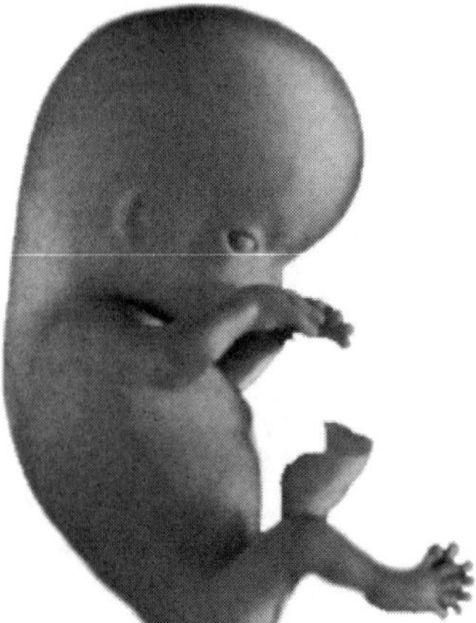

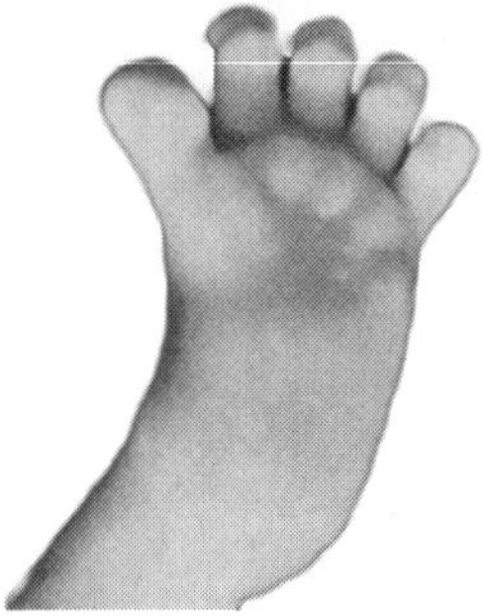

Thoughts:

....

....

DAY 59

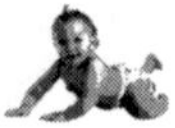

The sex of the fetus still can't be determined from visual inspection as the external genitalia are similar in appearance; this will change in a few days. The intestines are still located mostly in the umbilical cord. The baby can be seen grasping the umbilical cord, its other hand and its feet.

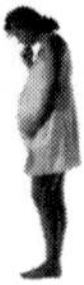

Sympathetic Pregnancy - If your spouse is starting to gain weight, feel queasy and vomit he may be experiencing Couvade Syndrome. These symptoms start around the end of the first trimester and increase in severity until birth. The suspected cause of these sympathetic pregnancy-like symptoms is psychological. The cure for this syndrome is the birth of the baby.

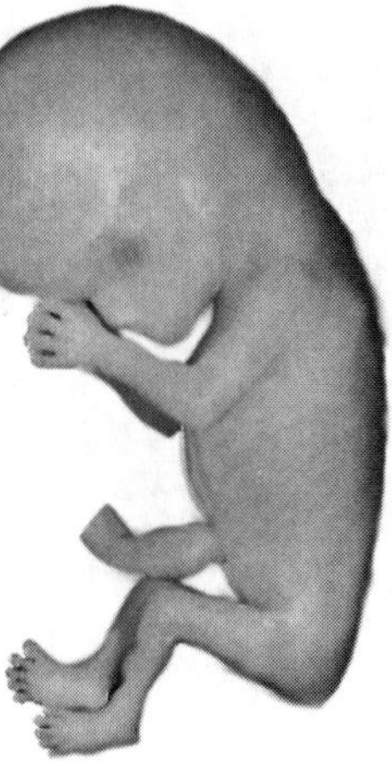

Notes:

....

....

DAY 60

The baby's head is over one-half the entire length of the body. Fingerprints are present on the fingers. The fingers will close around small objects placed in the baby's hand. Fingernails are just starting to grow and will reach the tips of the fingers by Week 32.

Swelling and leg cramps are common. Standing too long, getting tired and not eating the right foods can make these cramps more frequent and severe. Getting enough calcium by drinking milk will reduce the likelihood of cramping.

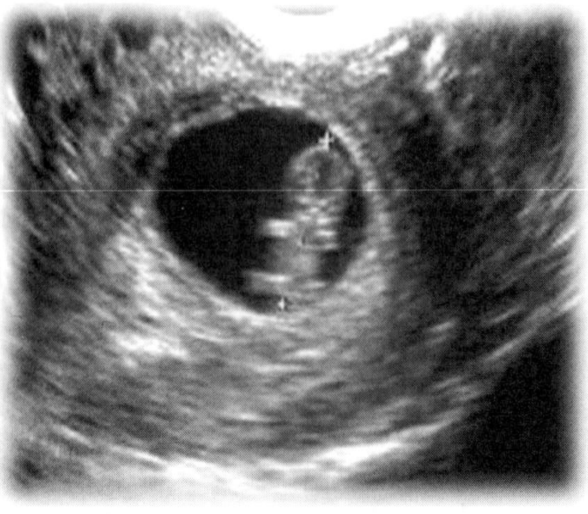

Thoughts:

....

....

DAY 61

The genitalia are beginning to take either male or female shape. If there is testosterone present, the genitalia will develop into a penis; otherwise, it will develop female. The eyes are open, but will again be shut as the eyelids develop and temporarily fuse until Week 26. Adrenal glands, which rest atop the kidneys, are formed and functional. Secreting hormones such as corticosteroids, androgens and estrogen derivatives that will have an organizing effect on the development of the brain and body that will make the physiological differences between male and female.

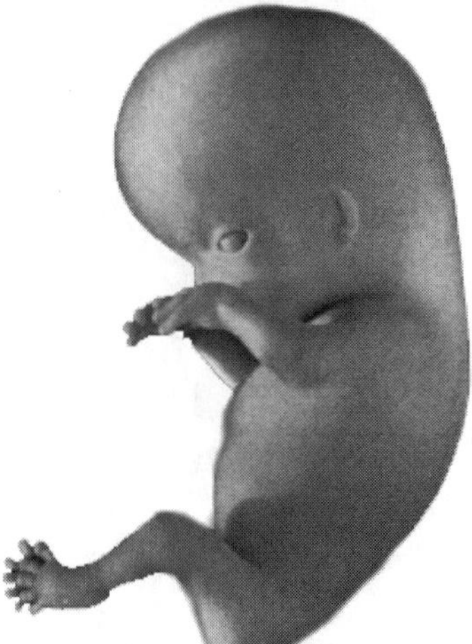

Notes:

....

....

DAY 62

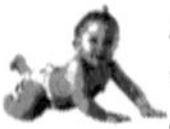

A touch of the lower torso causes an integrated reflex in which the arms are pulled up and the hips swivel sideways. The chin is well-defined, as are the fingers, with the beginnings of fingernails. The cranial nerves that move the eyes are going through rapid growth. The eye and the optic nerve are actually outgrowths of the forebrain. About this time the intestines start a period of rapid growth - reaching a length of 20-ft in the adult. The large and small intestine are visibly similar at this stage.

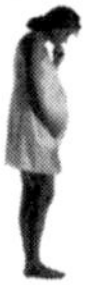

Your body is storing any excess iron you ingest in your liver. Although nearly 20% of all pregnant women experience iron deficiency anemia, it usually isn't until the 20th Week that your baby's iron needs can deplete your reserve.

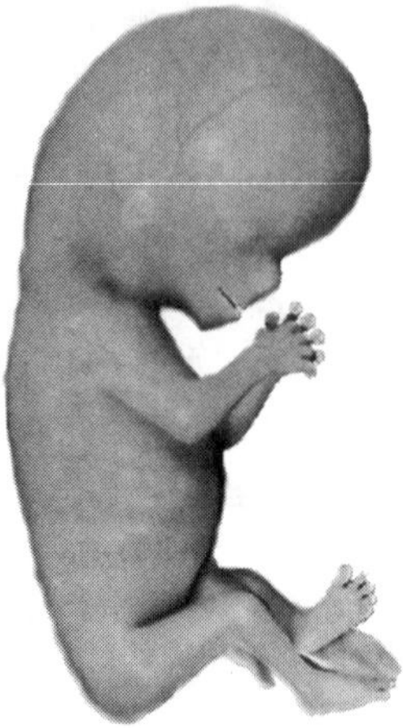

Thoughts:

....

....

DAY 63

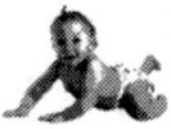

Parts of the brain involved in balance and coordination are establishing connections with the rest of the brain. The spinal cord is becoming anatomically mature, preparing for reflex movement. The baby will show bursts of motion with graceful stretching and rotational movements of the legs, arms and head. These movements, however, are still generated in the spinal cord. In a male, the urogenital folds fuse to form the penis and scrotum. In a female, the urogenital folds do not fuse, forming the labia minora while the labiogenital fold becomes the labia majora.

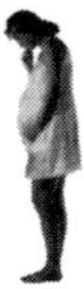

Your gums may be swollen, red and may bleed easily. These changes are a side-effect of the increased levels of pregnancy hormones. Good dental hygiene will minimize the risk of permanent damage.

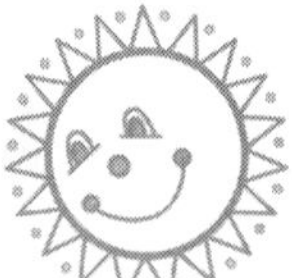

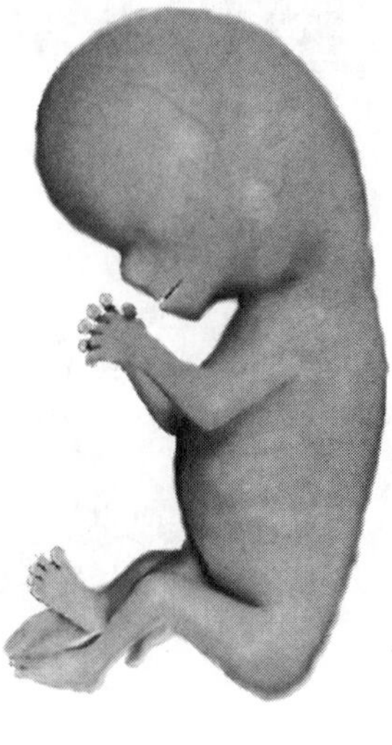

DAY 64

Behind the closed eyelids the cornea of the eye forms. However, the iris of the eye will not reflexively respond to light until the 8th month. Specific types of olfactory (sense of smell) neurons - those that are involved in detecting the presence of chemical substances - have formed and have a mature anatomical appearance.

Baby is 2-1/2 inches ❦ 1/2 oz.

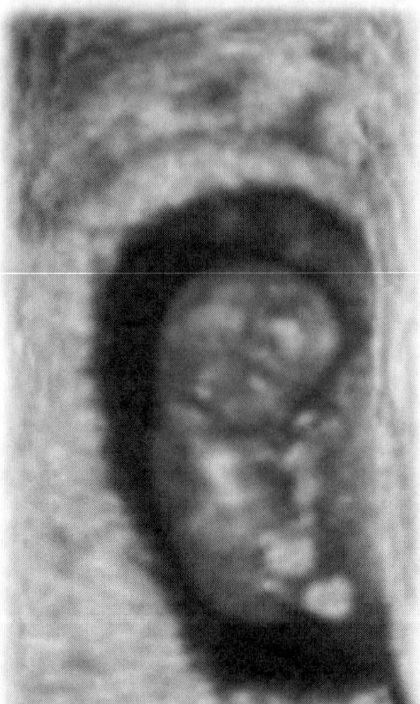

DAY 65

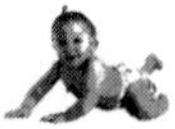

Brain waves originating from the deepest parts of the brain stem have been recorded in 10 week old embryos. The significance of this brain electrical activity is unknown and there are no cyclical changes in the type of recorded brain waves as would be seen during sleep/wake cycles in older fetuses. The spinal vertebrae in the neck and upper chest start to harden.

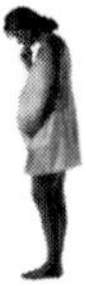

Fullness and heightened sensitivity of the breasts occurs now. Areolas and nipples become more pigmented and tender. On average a woman's breasts will enlarge 1-2 cup sizes during the course of the pregnancy, and will account for about 10% of her total weight gain (about 3 lbs.).

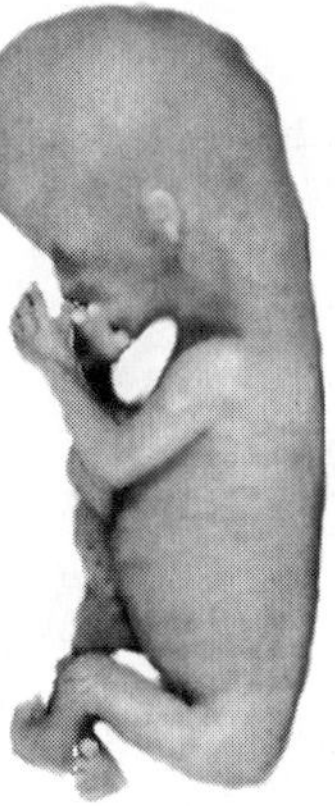

Notes:

....

....

DAY 66

The baby will show hand-to-head movements, as well as hand-to-face and hand-to-mouth movements. The kidneys - which formed in Week 5 - have migrated into the back of the abdominal cavity. The kidneys have been functioning for two weeks, producing urine which the baby excretes into the amniotic fluid.

You will gain about a pound per week between your 4th and 7th month of pregnancy. You've probably gained a couple of pounds by now; most of the weight is due to increased blood volume.

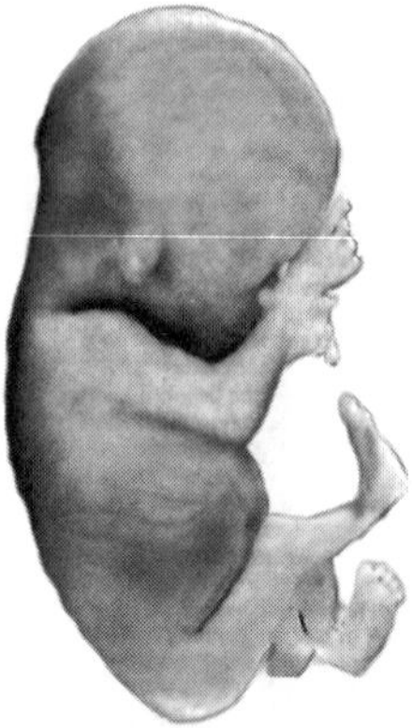

Thoughts:

....

....

DAY 67

Since the mouth area has such a large representation in the brain there are lots of mouth openings and closing now, and integrated swallowing of amniotic fluid. What does it taste like? Your baby can't taste anything yet, as taste function is still a few weeks away. Tooth buds for the milk teeth are present in the jaw and buds for the permanent teeth are positioned just to the inside of the baby teeth.

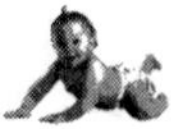

As your pregnancy progresses you'll notice the darkening of the vertical line that extends from your navel to the top of your pubic area. This is the linea alba (white line) which will darken into linea nigra under the influence of increased melanin.

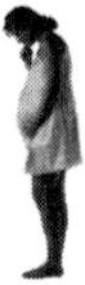

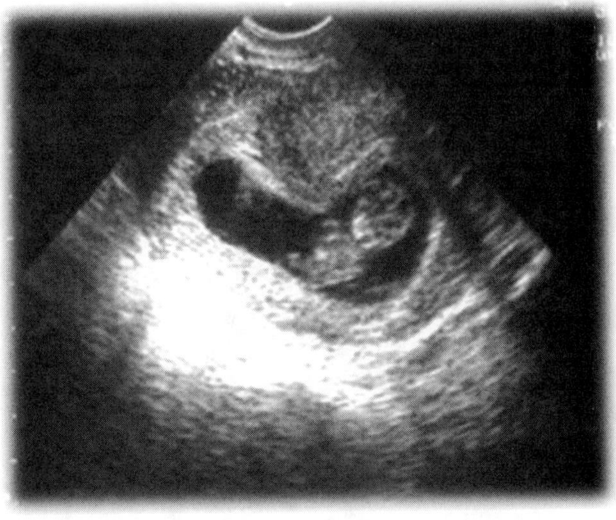

DAY 68

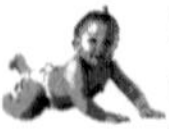

If your baby were to experience warmer or colder temperatures, it would react to them now. The sensitivity of the skin to touch matures in a very defined sequence or pattern, with the areas most sensitive in the adult developing first. The mouth area is already responsive and now the genital area responds to touch. The last area to be sensitive will be the back.

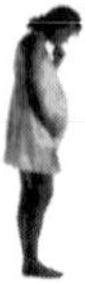

Your face can be affected by increased melanin as blotches of pigmentation appear on the forehead and cheeks. This is commonly known as the 'mask of pregnancy' and will disappear after birth.

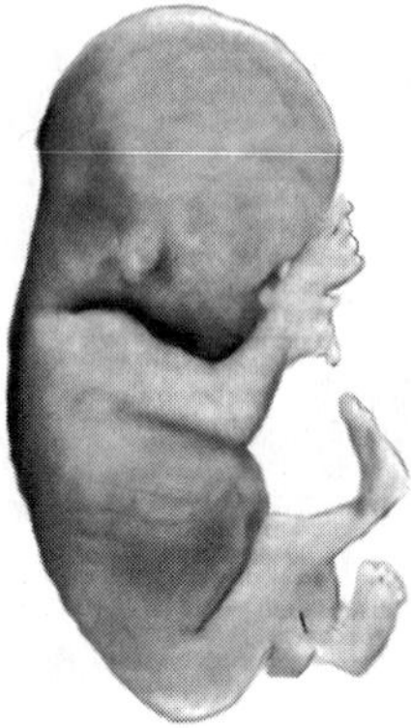

Thoughts:

....

....

DAY 69

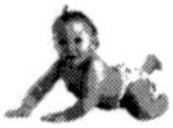

Your baby can squint and wrinkle the skin on its forehead, showing that the facial muscles and their control by the brain are functional. The voice box (larynx) is forming, although the baby can't make any sounds in the fluid-filled womb because of the absence of air. However, some doctors have reported crying-like sounds in nonviable babies exposed to air at 16 - 18 weeks gestation.

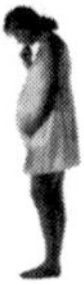

Drink plenty of fluids to keep adequately hydrated. The amniotic fluid is replaced every 3 to 4 hours so you need to maintain fluids. Keep a water bottle with you when you leave the house for extended periods.

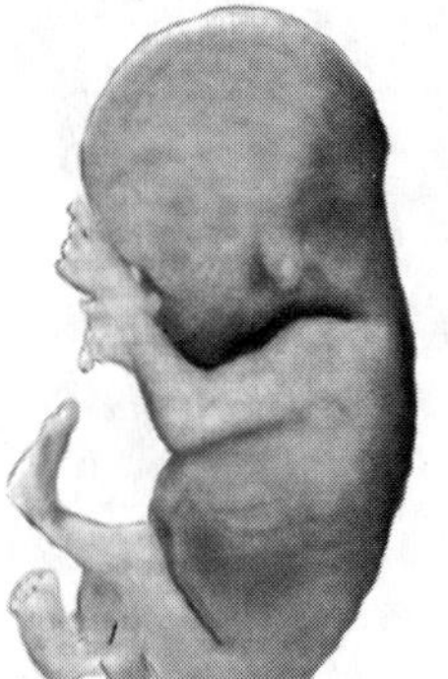

Notes:

....

....

DAY 70

The uterus has now doubled in size from the pre-pregnancy state to accommodate the growing baby. Your baby will stretch out and show breathing-like movements and lots of jaw openings and closings.

The placenta will become a major producer of the hormones that will sustain the pregnancy and some of those that will be necessary for milk production after the baby is born.

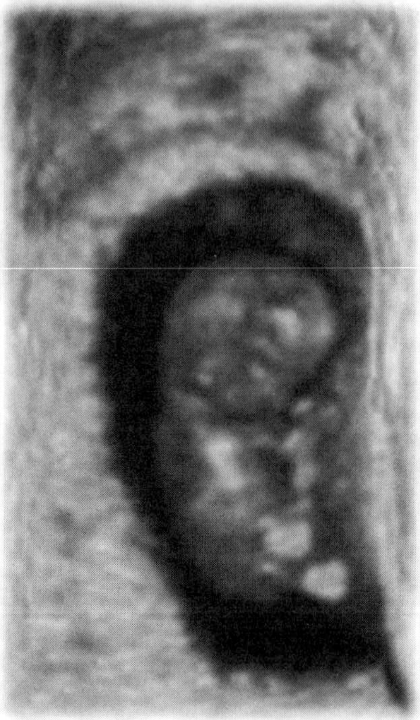

DAY 71

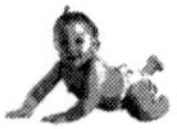

Breathing-like movements are observed in ultrasound recordings. The rib cage is forming to protect the internal organs. The liver is now manufacturing bile which will aid in the digestion of dietary fats later on. As a reference, the baby is now about the same size as a lime.

Baby is 3 inches ❦ 3/4 oz.

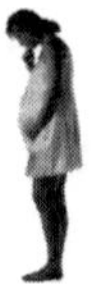

Hemorrhoids can be an unpleasant experience during pregnancy. Drink lots of fluids, eat fresh fruits and vegetables. Take walks, and don't sit in one place for too long to minimize their frequency and severity.

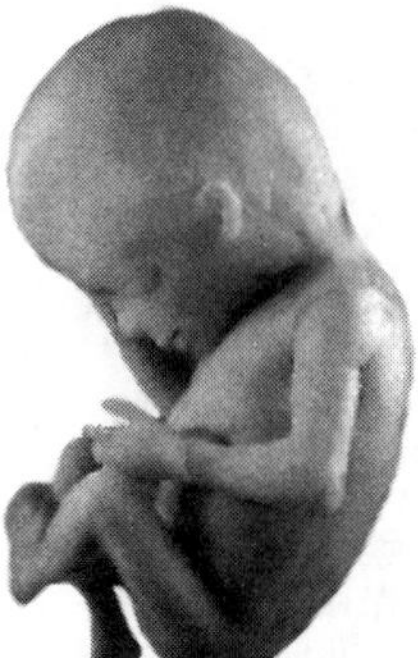

Notes:

....

....

DAY 72

Yawns can be observed during some ultrasound examinations. Myelination is occurring in neurons and nerves at a fast rate. Animal studies have shown that the speed at which a neural signal travels through the nervous system increases as the animal matures - due mostly to the efficient signal conduction properties of myelin. Myelin enables nerve signals to be relayed from one region to another and plays a role in the coordination and complexity of behavior.

Too much caffeine can be harmful to the baby-- how much is too much is not exactly known. Studies suggest that 3 cups of coffee per day (300 mg caffeine) can affect the baby's birth weight. Caffeine may decrease blood flow through the placenta, depriving the baby of oxygen and nutrients.

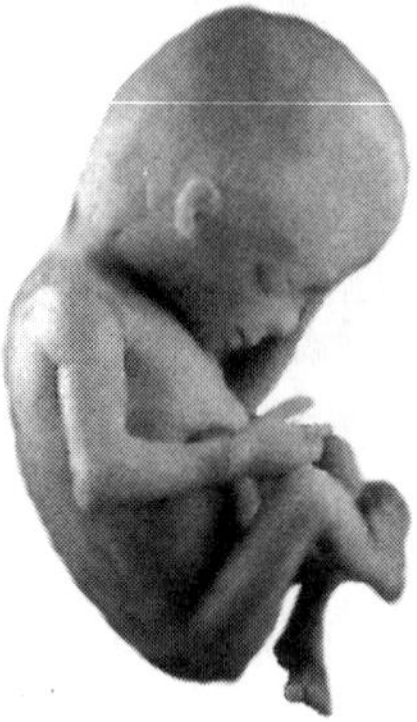

Thoughts:

....

....

DAY 73

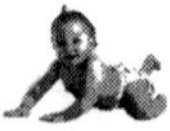

Muscle movements are becoming coordinated and spontaneous. For example, a hand to the mouth is self-initiated and may be an indication of purposeful behavior. In other words, your baby acts as if it "wants" to do it. The neural pathway from the cerebral cortex through the internal capsule to the spinal cord generates this observed behavior.

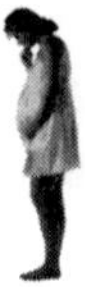

Estimated due dates are just that - estimates. Since calculations are based on a 28-day menstrual cycle, women who have shorter or longer cycles may deliver earlier or later than their estimated due date. As your pregnancy progresses, your doctor or midwife will reassess your due date using ultrasound tests, uterine size and heartbeat detection measurements.

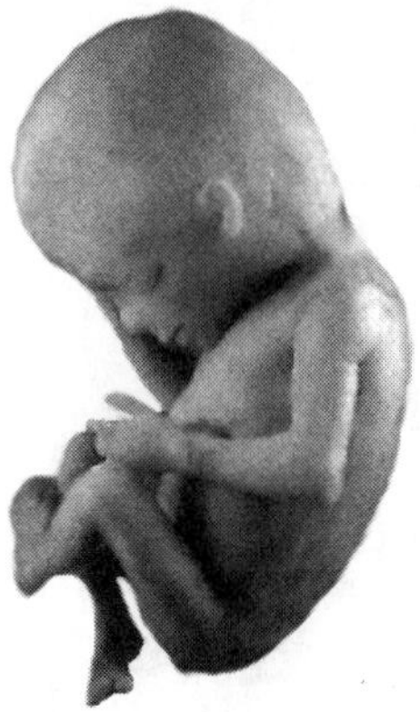

Notes:

....

....

DAY 74

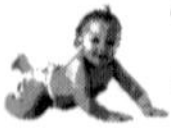

The tongue has mature taste buds now. Taste buds are more concentrated along the tongue and mouth cavity than they are in the adult. As your baby grows through childhood and adolescence, the taste buds spread out over the tongue and are distributed over a wider surface area. Can this anatomy explain why some foods appear to taste differently to kids?

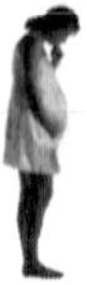

Sinus headaches are a common complaint during early pregnancy. Remember that over-the-counter drugs including aspirin, acetaminophen, ibuprophin and decongestants should be avoided unless directed by your doctor.

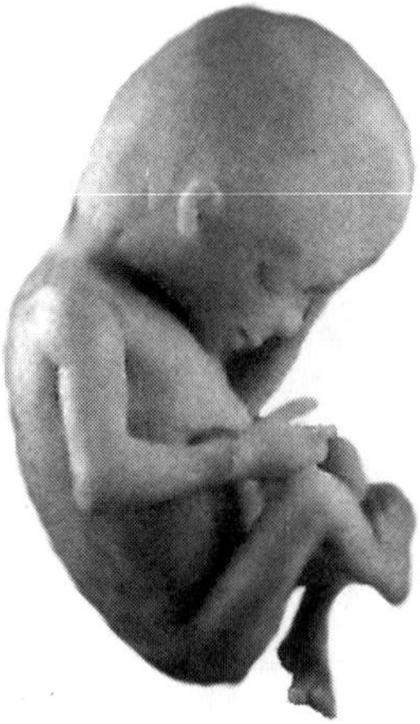

Thoughts:

....

....

DAY 75

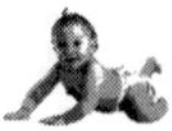

The sense of smell starts to develop now. Smell, or the olfactory sense, is complex and has several distinct systems that detect substances not just in the air. The baby is exposed to a rich environment of odors and tastes in the amniotic fluid. Researchers have found over 390 distinct compounds in amniotic fluid. The salivary glands are formed but won't secrete saliva until Week 16.

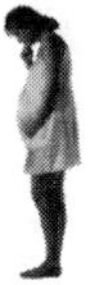

It's never too early to start thinking about a name. The back-and-forth decision making process that occurs when selecting a name keeps everyone involved and a part of the pregnancy.

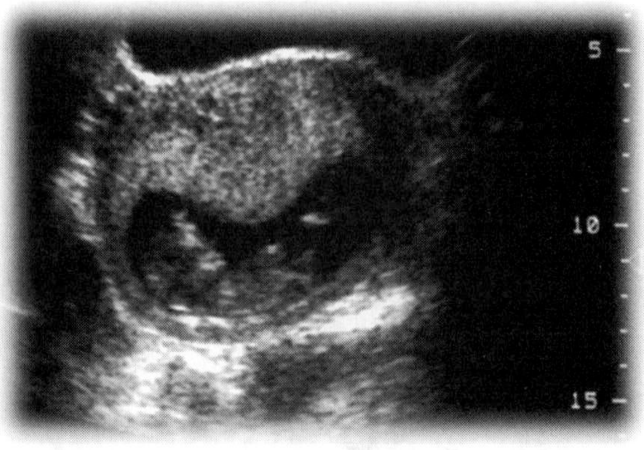

Notes:

....

....

DAY 76

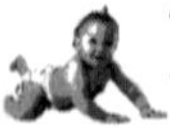

The skull bones are formed, growing and hardening. The various skull bone plates grow by adding new bone to the external surface of the bone and actively removing existing bone from the inside of the skull cavity. The effect is an outward expansion of the curved skull bones to make room for the growing brain.

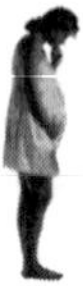

Leg cramps are common in calf muscles. The cramp, or Charley Horse, can be caused by not enough calcium and/or too much phosphorus in your diet. Drink more milk, cut down on processed foods that contain added phosphates. To alleviate a leg cramp sit with the leg outstretched, slowly bend your upper body toward your foot and flex the foot.

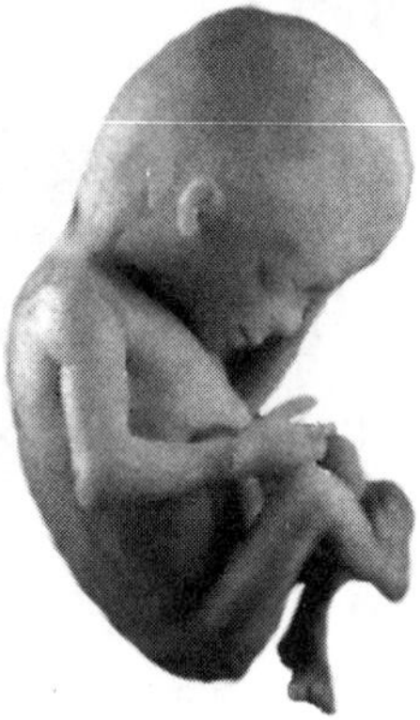

Thoughts:

....

....

DAY 77

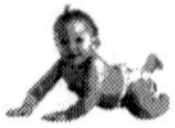

The olfactory nerve (smell) reaches the brain and provides chemoreceptive information to the brain. The olfactory system is now mature enough to be capable of detecting substances. Bone marrow is now producing blood and will be the only region to do so after birth. The liver and spleen only produce blood prenatally. Fetal blood doesn't coagulate until now.

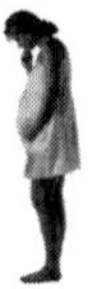

Your teeth can be affected by the hormonal changes of pregnancy. Inflammation of the gums (gingivitis) can develop as well as small sores called 'pregnancy tumors.' These afflictions will go away after birth. Dentists recommend that you get your teeth cleaned at the end of the second trimester (around 25 weeks).

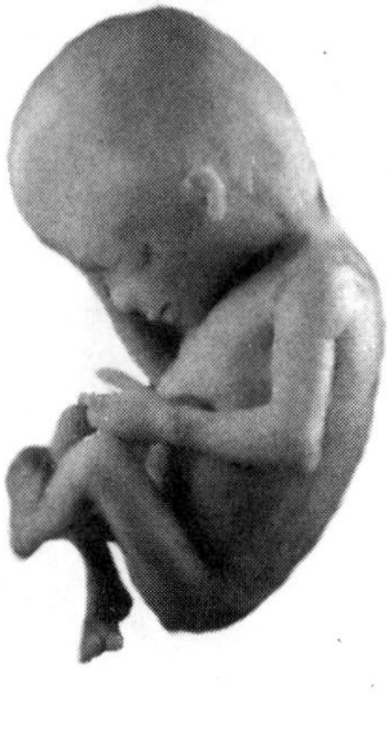

Notes:

....

....

DAY 78

The baby's mouth shows spontaneous movement including the lips opening and closing. The taste buds are present and the neural fibers relaying taste information to the brain are in place. The baby can also swallow and taste amniotic fluid. Amazing studies have demonstrated that 12-week old babies prefer sweet over sour substances injected into the amniotic fluid. Assuming that increased swallowing indicates preference, scientists have shown that injecting sweet-tasting substances like sucrose into amniotic fluid increase swallowing while injecting sour substances decrease the rate of swallowing.

Baby is 3-1/2 inches ❦ 1 oz.

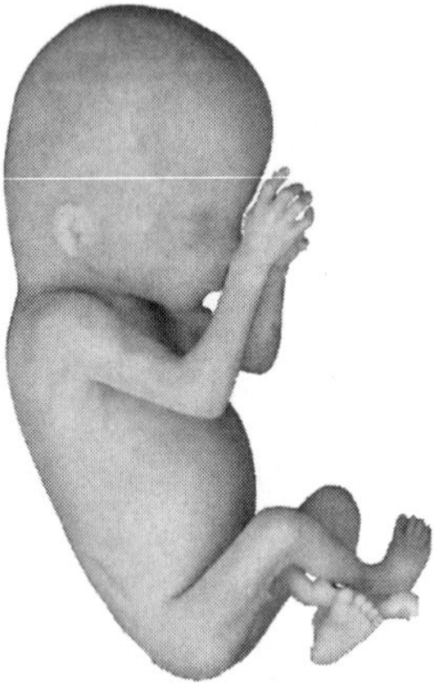

Thoughts:

....

....

DAY 79

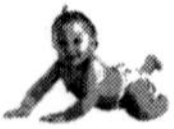

In an interesting series of studies, observations of babies at 12 weeks shows that they not only suck their thumbs but that they also show a preference for the right or left thumb! Babies observed at later periods - 20, 28, 30, and 34 weeks - also showed a preference for one thumb over the other. Just like in adults, about 90% of the fetuses preferred their right thumb--suggesting that they were right-handed. The significance of this finding is that lateralization of brain function (reflected in right or left-handedness) appears to occur very early. Just so you know...the fetuses that sucked their right thumb did become right-handed later in life.

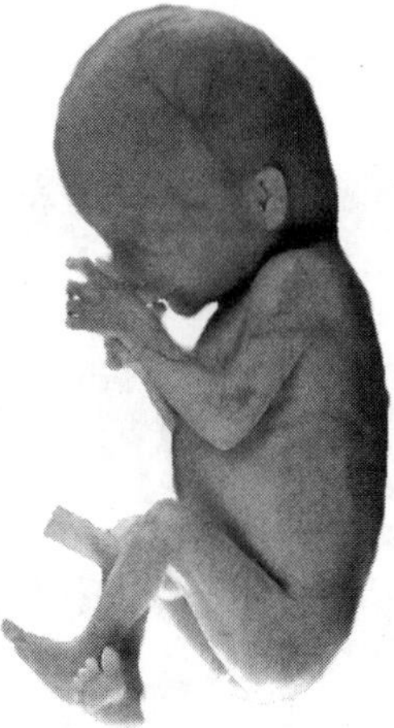

Notes:

....

....

DAY 80

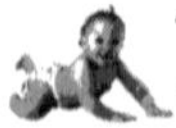

The baby can show 'startle-like' movements to loud sounds even though the auditory system is not functioning yet. Some researchers think that the touch receptors in the skin, specifically Pacinian corpuscles which respond to deep pressure, may be responsible for these early sensorimotor responses. The baby's response to sound takes a second or two after the loud noise. You have probably felt sound waves too, like the low frequency thump of a bass drum.

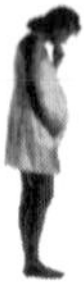

You'll need a steady supply of Vitamin C to help build your baby. 80 - 100 mg per day is recommended. In addition to citrus juices such as orange juice, many vegetables like broccoli and green bell peppers are high in Vitamin C. Eating just one orange will give you 70 mg Vitamin C.

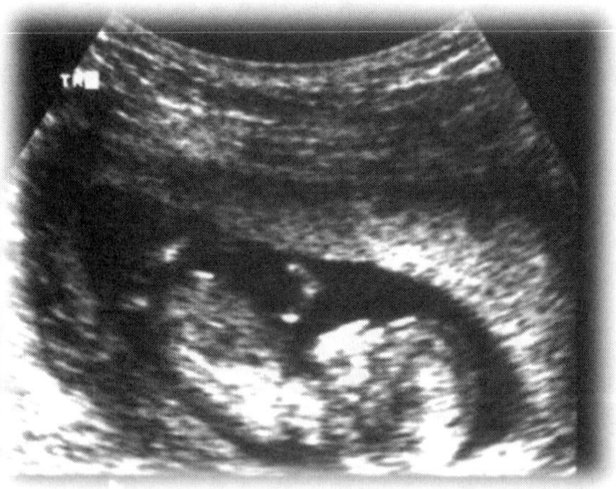

DAY 81

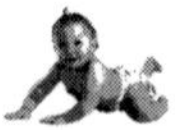

Touching the baby along the back generates a response that includes the mouth opening and the corners of the mouth turn up, and the chest and abdominal muscles tightening to elevate the rib cage and flatten the abdominal wall. All these movements are characteristic of a ticklish response. The baby can turn its head from side-to-side, and will move the head even more as the neck lengthens in the next few weeks. The baby can raise and lower its eyebrows.

Babies have many bone segments that grow independently and then fuse to become one complete bone. A baby has 305 bones that will be reduced in number to the 206 bones that adults have. For example, the skull is made of up 8 distinct bones in a baby - these will fuse into one cohesive bone in the adult.

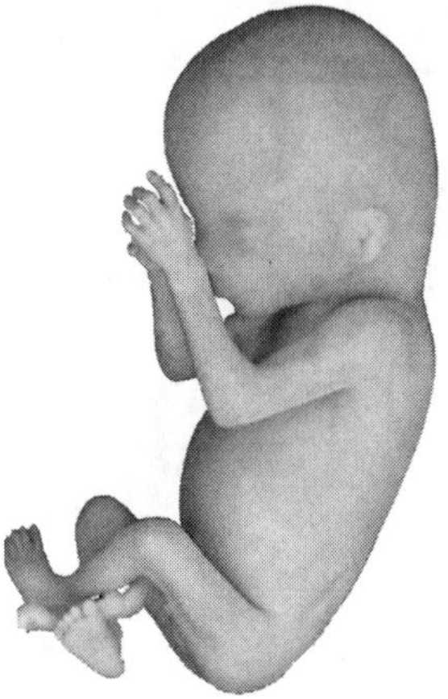

Notes:

....

....

DAY 82

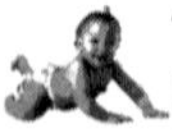

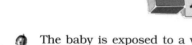

The baby is exposed to a very noisy uterine environment. Between the sounds of the mother's heart beating, blood rushing through the umbilical cord and your digestive churning and movement, the sound intensity level varies between 72 and 96 dB. For a reference, normal speaking voice registers 60 - 70 dB. The cerebellum, which controls muscle coordination and some autonomic activity, is formed.

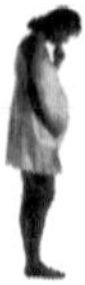

Protein is a very important nutritional need as it provides amino acids which are the building blocks of the cells of the body. At least eight ounces per day of eggs, meats, fish and dairy products should provide enough protein for you and your developing baby.

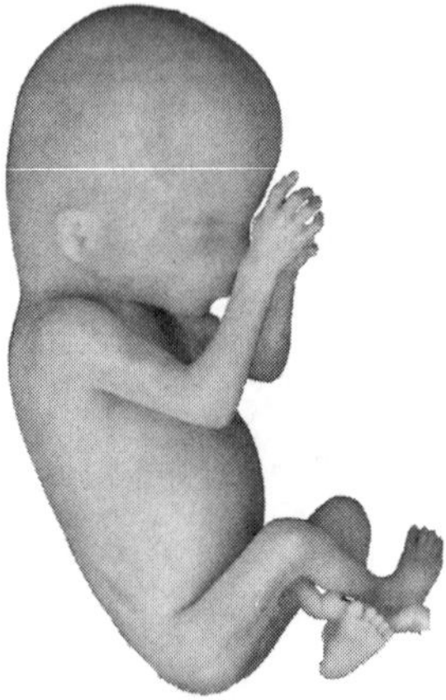

Thoughts:

....

....

DAY 83

The ovaries are formed and on the move in the female's abdomen. The testes in the male are positioned at about the level of the leg-hip socket and will slowly descend into the scrotum by Week 32.

Summary of Movements Observed to Date

Any movement	7 weeks
Startle	8
Hiccups	8
Isolated arm movements	9
Head tilted back	9
Hand-face contact	10
Breathing-like movements	10
Jaw opening	10
Stretching	10
Head tilted forward	10
Yawn	11
Suck and swallow	12

from deVries et al. (1982)

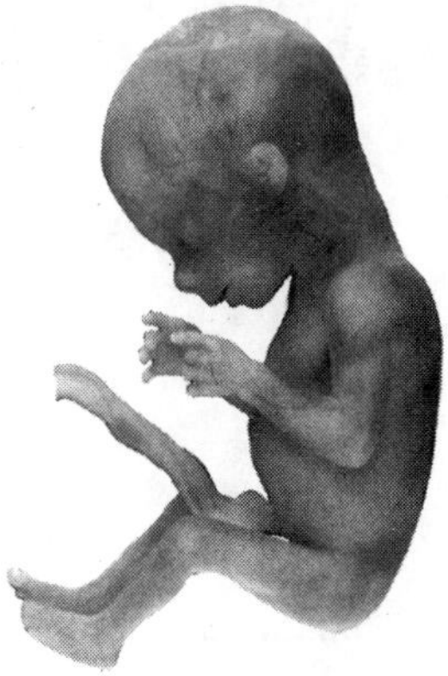

DAY 84

Shown below is a baby attached to its placenta and chorionic membranes by the umbilical cord. Look at the arms...the upper arm and lower arm appear to be properly proportioned now. The legs still have some catching up to do until they are properly proportioned. The spontaneous activity levels of the baby are quite high, however the baby is still too small for these movements to be felt by you.

Today is the end of the first trimester (3 month period) of your pregnancy.

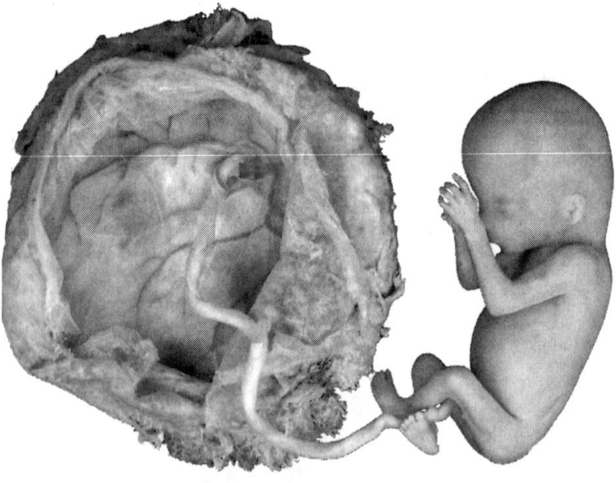

Thoughts:

....

....

DAY 85

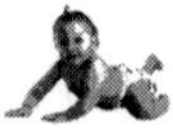

The mouth is highly developed and many of the components are fully formed and functioning. For example, the taste buds are present and the salivary glands are functional. The baby doesn't need these yet but behavioral responses to taste cues can be detected now.

Baby is 4 inches ❦ 1-3/4 oz.

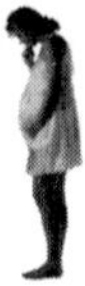

Today begins the 4th month of your pregnancy...the Second Trimester. This month's checkup will involve weight and blood pressure, urine sample, fetal heartbeat detection, measurement of the size and shape of your uterus and a general exam.

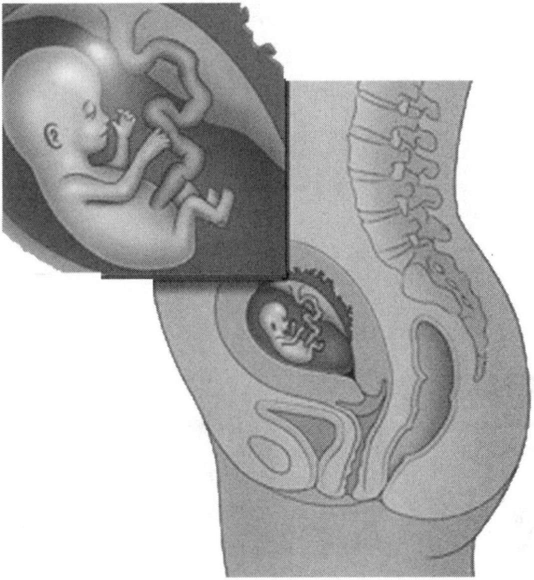

Notes:

....

....

DAY 86

The finger pads have regressed by now. Your baby's hands look just like yours now, except in miniature form, about the size of your fingernail. Take a look at the changes that have occurred in a few weeks in the shape of your baby's hands and fingers. Notice how the tissue between the fingers at 7 weeks has disappeared by 13 weeks. This dying-away of tissue is an example of programmed cell death that helps shape and refine the body. Cell death is especially important in determining the final anatomical structure of the brain.

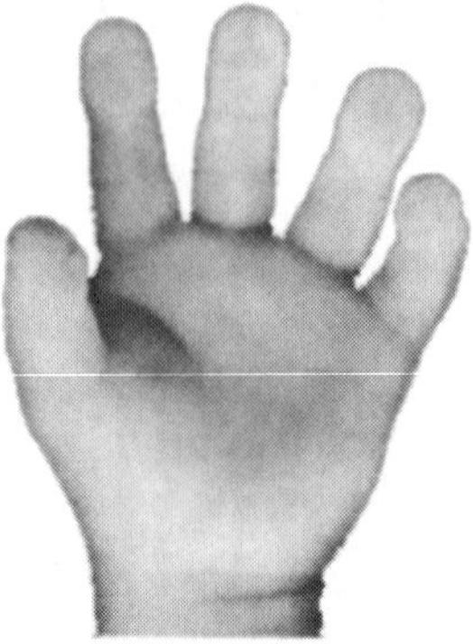

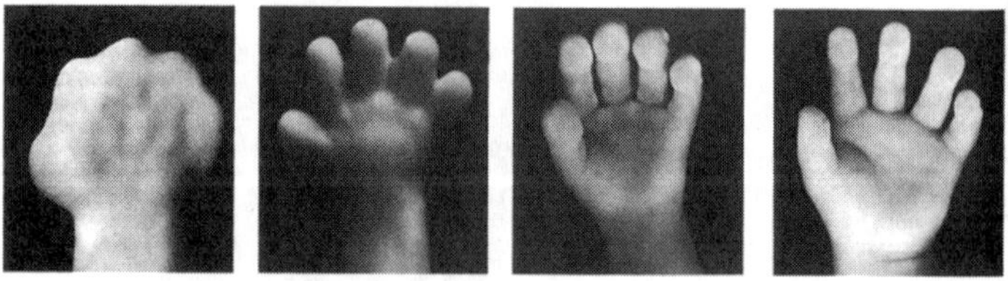

6 weeks *7 weeks* *8 weeks* *13 weeks*

DAY 87

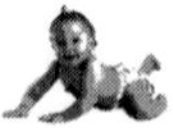

Behavioral responses are smooth and purposeful as muscular functioning is now fluid, coordinated and graceful. Some investigators have speculated that the fluid environment in the womb leads to an early, rapid maturation of coordinated muscle activity in this nearly weightless environment. Once the baby emerges outside, gravity takes over and the familiar uncoordinated, flopping and non-graceful movements of the newborn "out of its home environment" is seen....a fish out of water so to speak. Imagine if you had trained to be a sprinter on dry land and the track for the performance was ice; the change in the environment would negate most of your skill. Newborns, who have developed in an aquatic world and are introduced to a terrestrial one at birth, must re-adjust to their new environment.

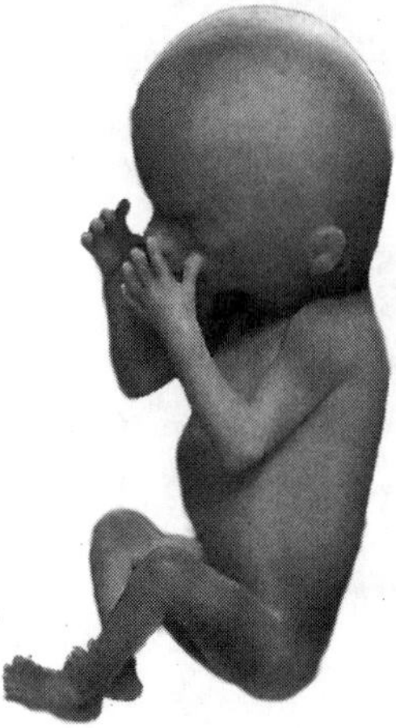

Notes:

....

....

DAY 88

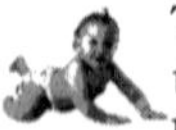

The spleen is producing red blood cells and is fully functional now. When viewed on a ultrasound, you can see your baby exert breathing-like movements and swallowing amniotic fluid. Both of these behaviors appear to be practice for air-breathing and eating. The ribs are developing now and will ossify over the next few weeks. The breast bone (sternum) hardens at Week 20.

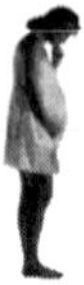

The hormonal changes in your body are becoming apparent. The areola (dark nipple portion of your breasts) may have darkened and gotten larger as well. Your uterus is now the size of a grapefruit.

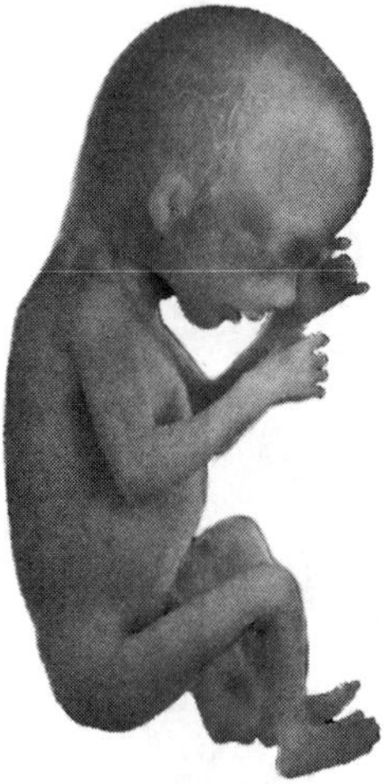

Thoughts:

....

....

DAY 89

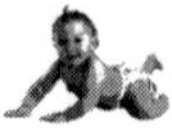

The neck is still growing, distancing the chin from the chest. Each of us has a unique patterning of hair on our scalp. Your baby's individual scalp hair pattern develops now, cow-licks and all. Sex hormones (testosterone and estrogen) are produced by the pituitary gland now. The entire repertoire of movements observed now is the same as that seen at birth.

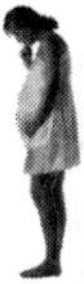

Changes in your vision are likely to occur. Because your eyes also retain fluid during pregnancy, the refractive angles between your lens and retina can change. When this happens light doesn't focus where it should on the retina and objects can appear blurry. Your vision will return to the way it was after your baby is born.

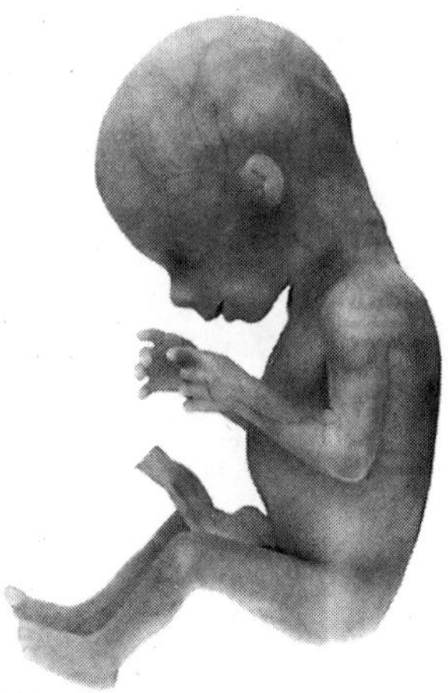

Notes:

....

....

DAY 90

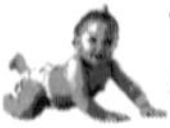

Touching the baby's palm causes the hand to close by the clenching of the ring finger and pinky. Sometimes the thumb clenches only briefly. The grasp is held for only a few seconds. This is a big change compared to about a month ago when the response was a quick flexion of the fingers that wasn't sustained for any period of time.

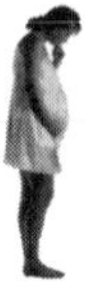

Exercise has many benefits for you during pregnancy and new research is showing that your baby benefits from your exercise too. Babies born to mothers who exercised during pregnancy are leaner at 5 years of age, tolerate stress better and have advanced neurobehavioral development.

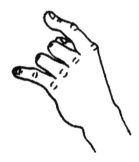

Hand at rest

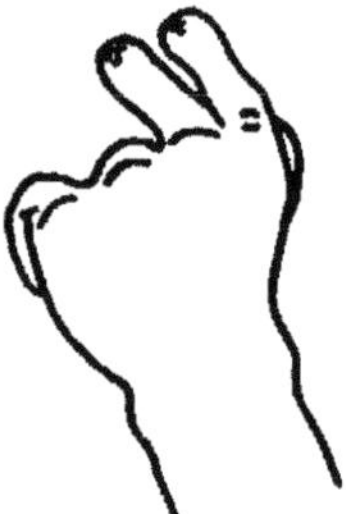

Grasping response to touch of palm

from Humphrey (1964).

Thoughts:

....

....

DAY 91

Your baby will now show integrated responses to outside stimulation. Studies have shown that touching the baby's lip area causes an early sucking reflex that's visible as a pursing of the lips. Other times the baby may turn away or toward the touch. The occurrence of these behaviors show that the underlying neural and muscular systems are functioning to produce these complex behaviors, complex because they involve, at a minimum: the sensation and perception of an external touch stimulus, the relaying of that information to the appropriate parts of the brain and the generation of an appropriate, adaptive neural response that moves the muscles to produce the observable behavior. Pretty amazing!

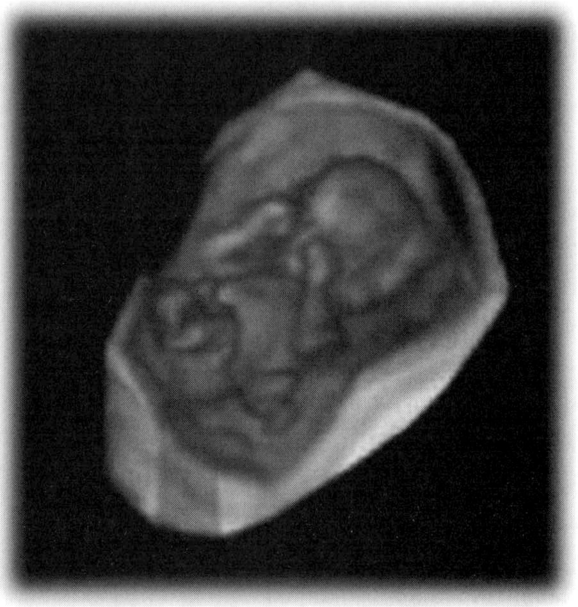

DAY 92

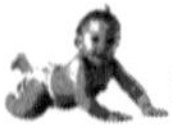

Believe it or not, your baby can actually grasp objects placed into its hand. Studies have demonstrated that a small wire placed in the baby's palm will elicit what is know as a "grasping reflex" where the fingers close around the object.

Baby is 4-1/2 inches ❦ 3 oz.

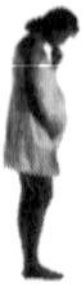

Scientists have shown that maternal sensitivity and affection have their roots in pregnancy. In other words, many mothers already love their babies - intensely - before they ever see them. Furthermore, the strength of those feelings increase throughout the pregnancy.

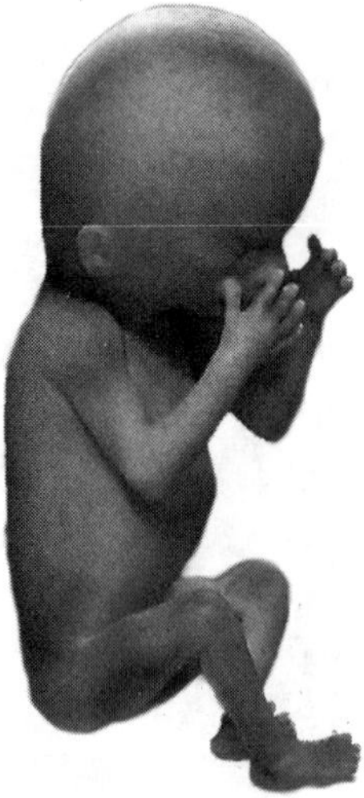

Thoughts:

....

....

DAY 93

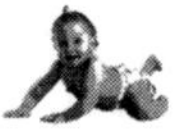

Up to now, the growth of the baby's head has been faster than that of the body. The body will now grow faster. All types of integrated movements occur: rolling from side to side, reaching for the cord, grasping the cord, swimming movements.

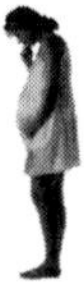

Questionnaires have been developed to measure a woman's attachment, relationship with, and feelings toward her baby. Women who report more attachment to their babies experienced more confidence in their new role as mother and showed better adjustment after the birth. Some of these items don't apply now because the baby is too small for you to feel its movements.

Prenatal Attachment Inventory

Factors	Sample items
Fantasy	I wonder what my baby looks like now I dream about the baby
Interaction	I know when my baby is asleep I can make my baby move
Affection	I feel love for the baby I enjoy feeling the baby move
Baby as distinct from self	I think my baby already has a personality I imagine calling baby by name
Sharing pleasures	I tell others what the baby is doing I let others put their hands on my belly

from Mueller (1993).

DAY 94

The taste buds are formed and the neural connections to the brain that relay taste information are functioning. Experiments have demonstrated that a bitter-tasting substance introduced into the amniotic fluid will cause the baby to behave as if the substance were tasted and a 'dislike' reaction evoked, complete with a facial expression.

Facial responses of newborns to various tastes. The early fetal responses described above are easily seen at birth.

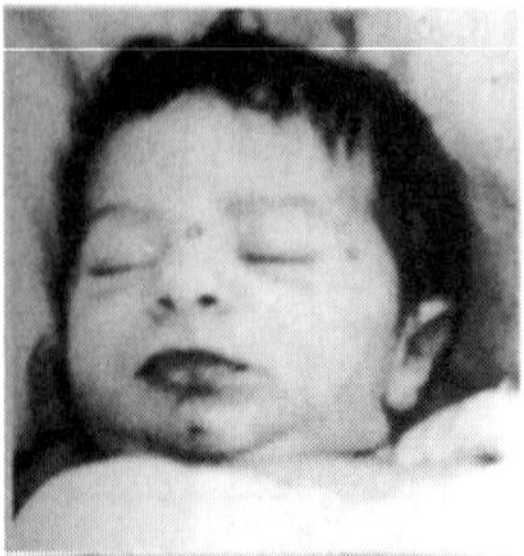

Sleeping baby

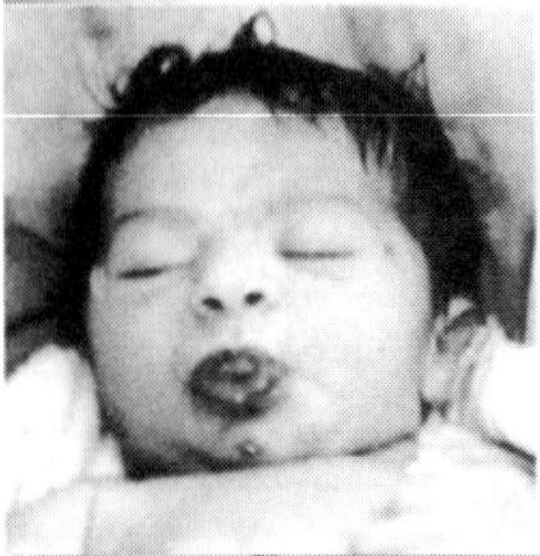

Sweet taste

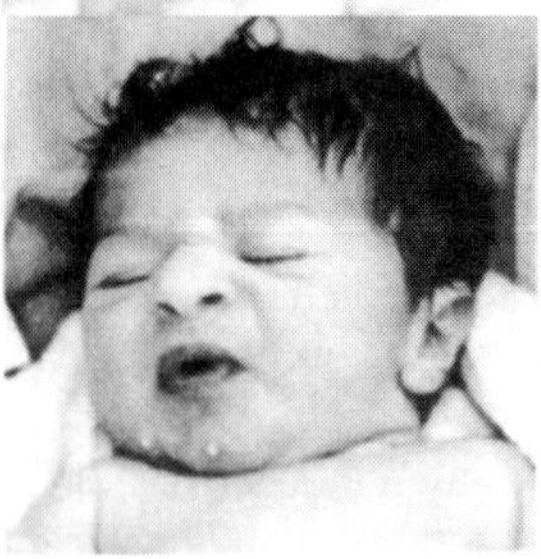

Bitter taste

from Baron, 1989.

DAY 95

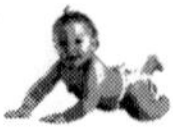

There is very fine hair on the head filling in the pattern of the scalp. Fingerprints are forming. Babies demonstrate what is known as the rooting reflex now. If they are stimulated/touched near the cheek they will turn their head toward the source...as if rooting or searching for a nipple.

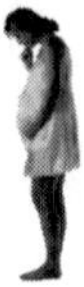

Depending on a number of factors your doctor may determine that prenatal tests of your baby are warranted. These tests are used to rule out the possibility of a problem. Amniocentesis involves taking a sample of the amniotic fluid around your baby and analyzing the contents of the fluid. This test is performed between 14 and 18 Weeks.

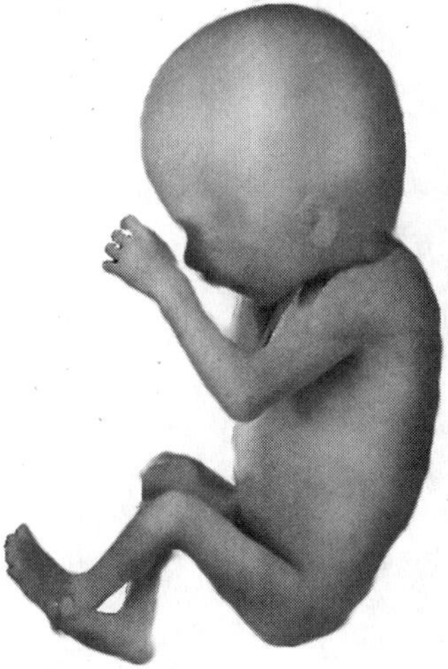

Notes:

....

....

DAY 96

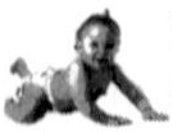

It is easy to differentiate a boy from a girl now as the external genitalia are distinct. The neck is clearly distinct from the shoulders. Swallowing of amniotic fluid is integrated and smooth. Toenails are growing. Slow, rolling eye movements are taking place behind the closed eyelids.

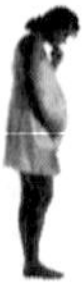

Another test is called the Alpha Feto Protein (AFP) test. A sample of blood is withdrawn from your arm and the sample is analyzed. High levels of AFP can indicate a problem. AFP tests are notorious for their registration of false positives - that is, indicating a problem when there is none. Typically a high AFP reading is followed up by additional tests such as amniocentesis and/or chorionic villus sampling.

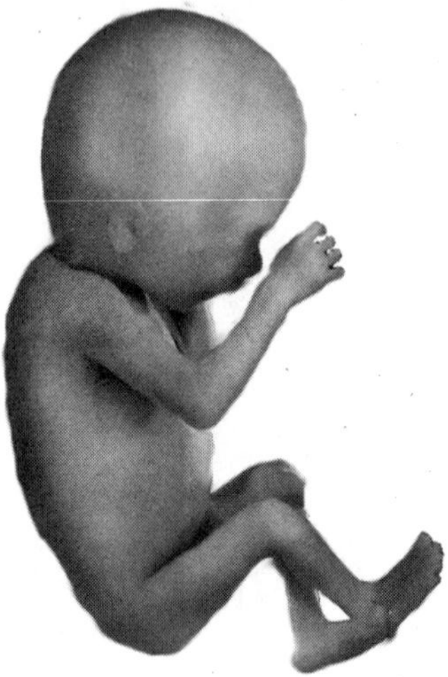

Thoughts:

....

....

DAY 97

The toe pads are starting to regress now and the foot looks just like a miniature version of your foot. You can see a heel, ankle and arch. Take a look at the progression of the foot in just a few weeks. The shape changed from a paddle-shaped flipper to a foot complete with distinct toes. Just as with the hand, the tissue between the toes, which gives a webbed appearance, dies away by the 14th week. The development of the foot lags about a week behind that of the hand.

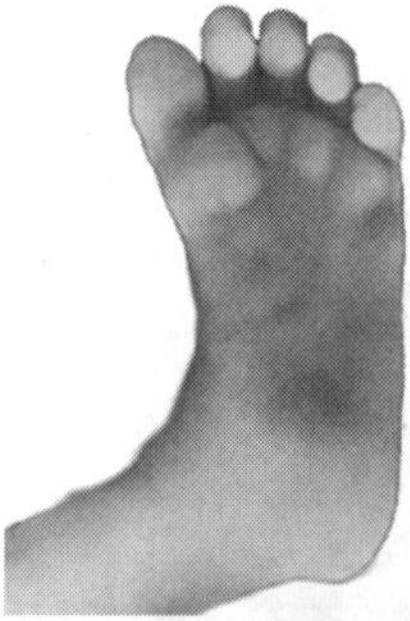

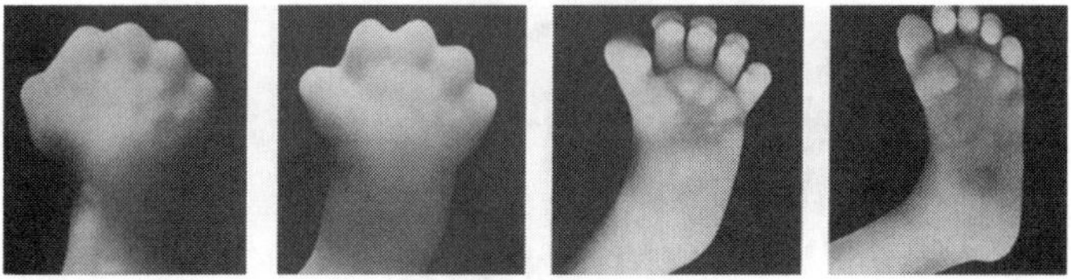

7 weeks *8 weeks* *9 weeks* *14 weeks*

Notes:

....

....

DAY 98

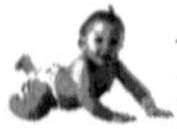

Amniotic fluid completely regenerates itself every three to four hours. Your baby is now producing urine and actually urinating into the amniotic fluid, making urine a large component of the amniotic fluid. Where the bulk of the amniotic fluid in general is made is not known. An analysis of amniotic fluid found over 390 distinct compounds. Some of these substances provide nutrition to your baby; others provide a rich sensory environment of tastes and chemical stimuli for your baby.

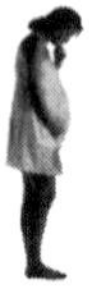

Iodine is necessary for proper thyroid gland function and nervous system development. Table salt is typically fortified with iodine. Vegetables and seafood have iodine as well.

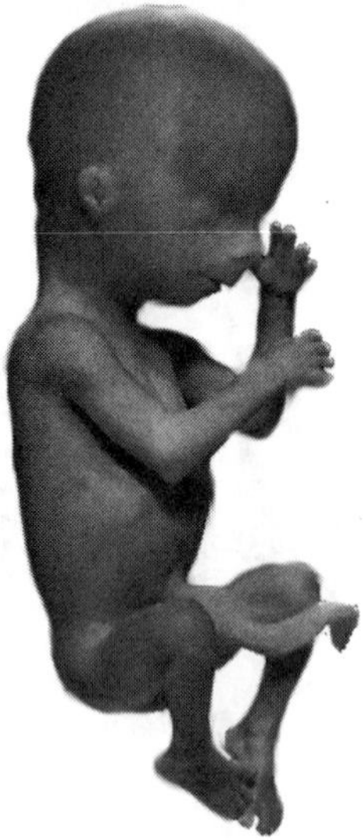

Thoughts:

....

....

DAY 99

Your baby may have developed the habit of sucking his or her thumb! You may even see your baby sucking its thumb if you have an ultrasound exam.

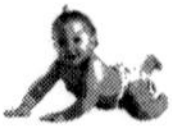

Baby is 5 inches ❦ 3-1/2 oz.

Chorionic villus sampling is a test that samples the finger-like projections (villi) of the developing placenta. The tissue sample is analyzed for chromosomal abnormalities and other birth defects.

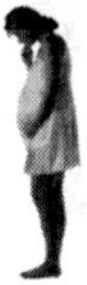

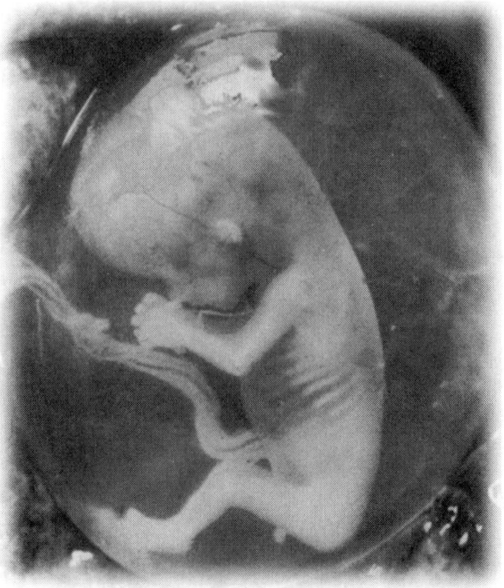

Notes:

....

....

DAY 100

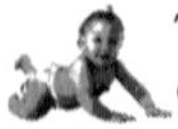

The skin has developed and is very thin. If the baby were outside you could clearly see blood vessels underneath the skin. The baby's entire torso - front and back - is sensitive to touch. And the heart is pumping about 100 pints of blood a day.

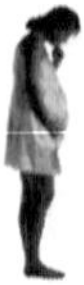

There is popular 'folklore' that a baby's heart rate can be used to predict the sex of the child: High heart rates (>140 bpm) mean a girl; heart rates below 140 bpm mean you're carrying a boy. This is just a myth. Baseline heart rate doesn't indicate the sex of the child. Some recent findings have shown a sex difference with girls having a slightly higher body temperature than boys. This measurement is obtained only under sensitive experimental conditions using complex monitoring equipment so don't count on learning your baby's body temperature before birth.

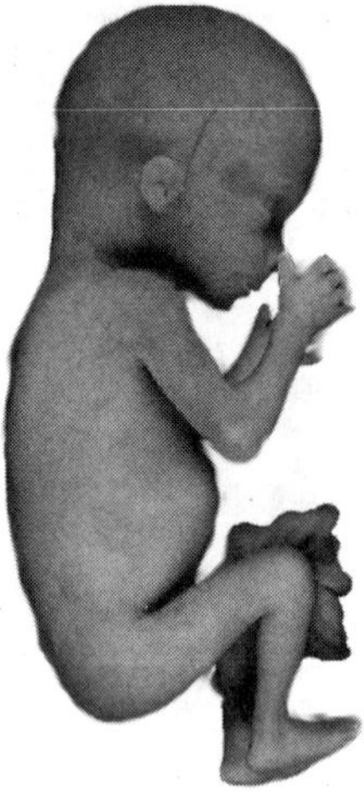

Thoughts:

....

....

DAY 101

Babies of this age will demonstrate individual differences in how they react to external stimulation. During amniocentesis procedures, ultrasound images are used to guide placement of the needle that samples the fluid. These records have shown a variety of responses by the baby to the needle/probe: some reach out and grab it, some turn away from it, some kick at it. Is this evidence for personality differences at this age?

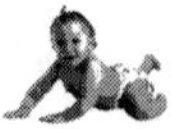

For some women, ginger capsules can reduce the symptoms of morning sickness. One study found that a 250-mg capsule of ginger each day reduced feelings of nausea in women experiencing severe symptoms. Ask your doctor before you take any remedies for morning sickness.

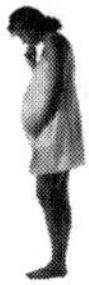

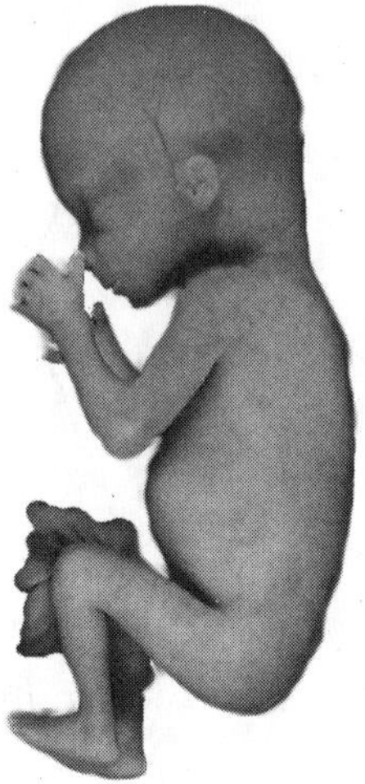

Notes:

....

....

DAY 102

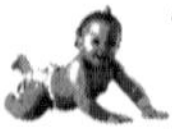

Touching the baby's palm now results in the ring and middle fingers (3rd and 4th) leading the clenching around the object. Next the index and pinky finger follow until all fingers are held tightly. The thumb flexes but does not wrap around or help secure the object yet.

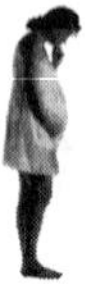

If your morning sickness hasn't subsided yet, it probably will soon. Most women feel their best during their 2nd trimester - energy levels return to near normal, the pregnancy is starting to show, and your complexion has a radiant glow.

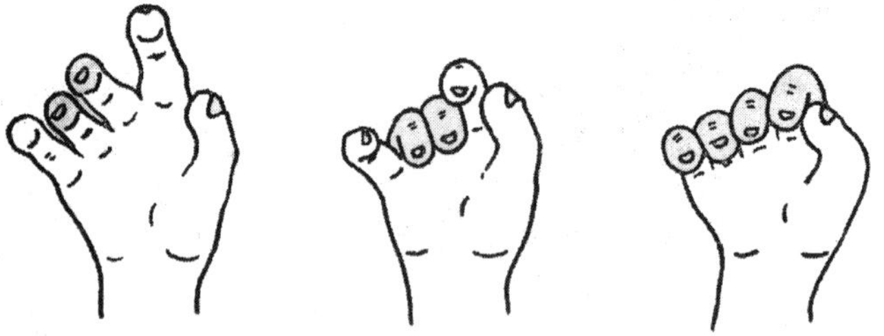

A. Hand at rest *B. 3rd & 4th fingers clench* *C. Index and pinky follow*

from Humphrey (1964).

Thoughts:

....

....

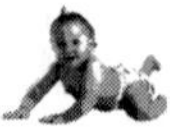

Real-time ultrasound images have shown that babies are very active now...some doing somersaults, others spinning in their fluid-filled environment. Why doesn't the umbilical cord get hopelessly tangled and knotted? Try bending a garden hose with high water pressure - the force of the blood rushing through the cord keeps it from kinking.

The development of arm posture starts with a flexion of the elbow at 12 Weeks, followed by flexion of the fingers at 20 Weeks and finally flexion of the wrist at 24 Weeks. Most systems develop along a near-to-far (proximal-distal) plan with regions closer to the trunk of the body maturing earlier. The arm follows a different plan.

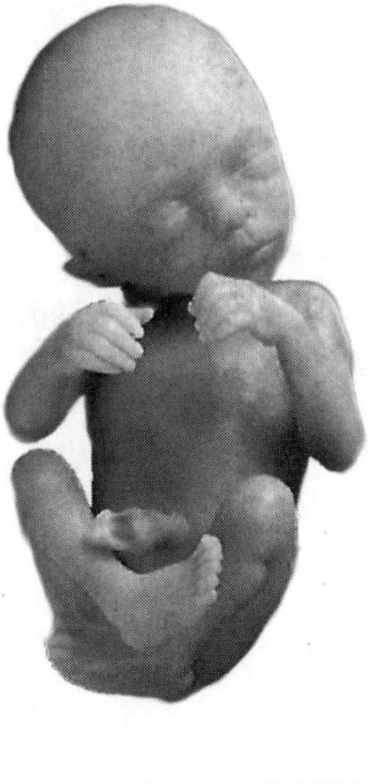

Notes:

....

....

DAY 104

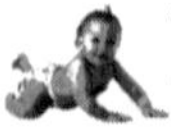

The insulating material known as myelin is forming around the nerves. These cells, made of fat, surround the axons or arms of the nerve and enable fast transmission of neural signals, while also preventing the signals in one axon from interfering with the activity in another. Myelin is similar to insulation on electrical wires - it prevents signals from getting crossed and helps information reach its intended target faster and more efficiently. Myelin will enable the appearance of more sophisticated, complex and integrated behaviors.

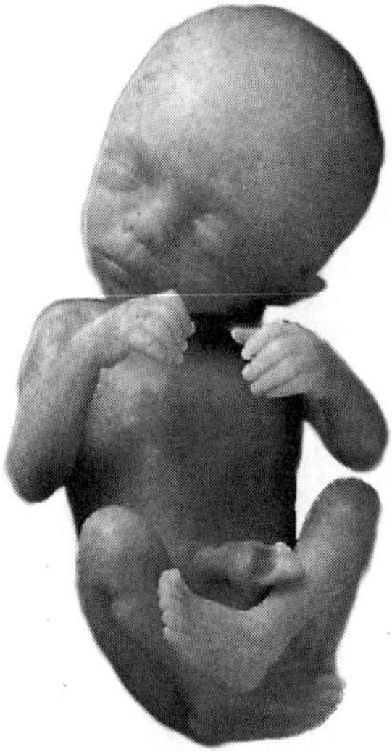

Thoughts:

....

....

DAY 105

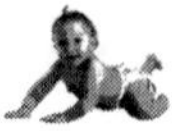

Many sensory systems (hearing, touch, taste, smell) and motor systems have appeared at this point...some have come online relatively early. For example, the ear was structurally complete at 8 weeks. The importance of myelin is that now these anatomical neural systems can start working without generating or receiving interference from other neighboring systems. The foundation of complex behaviors is in place because the neural wiring is in place.

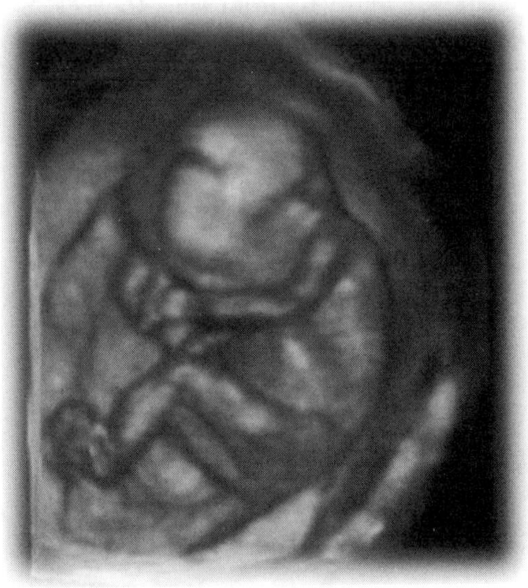

Notes:

....

....

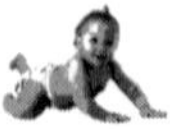

Seeing your baby hiccup is a common sight in real-time ultrasound examinations. The baby is practicing breathing using the amniotic fluid instead of air. All bone marrow generates new blood in the fetus. In the adult, only the ribs, breast bone, spinal vertebrae, thigh bone (femur), upper arm (humerus) and skull form new blood.

Baby is 5-1/2 inches ❦ 5 oz.

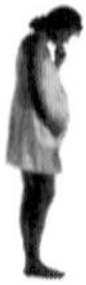

Your weight gain may vary from week-to-week. Some weeks you gain less than a pound, other weeks perhaps two pounds. This variability in week-to-week weight gain is normal.

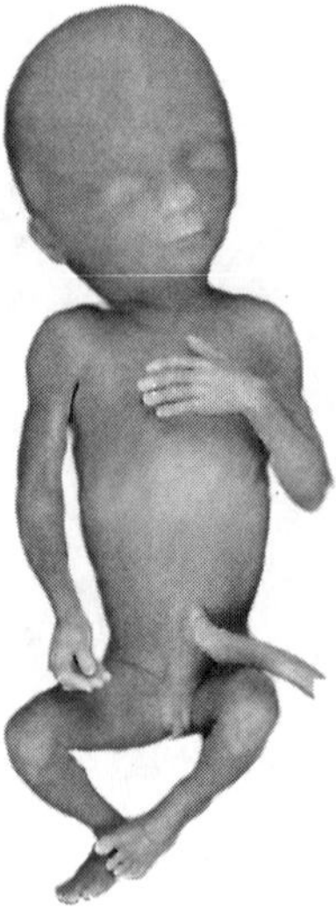

Thoughts:

....

....

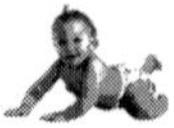

The baby's external genitalia are large enough and differentiated enough to be seen in an ultrasound image. Trained ultrasonographers can determine whether you're carrying a boy or girl now. If you have an ultrasound examination performed, be sure to indicate that you don't want to know the baby's sex until birth (if that's the case). The technician may inadvertently blurt out the sex or refer to the image as 'he' or 'she' if they assume you either want to know or already know the sex. Be clear in your instructions so that you aren't disappointed.

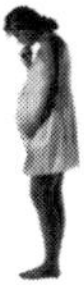

Until about Week 20, your placenta weighs more than the baby.

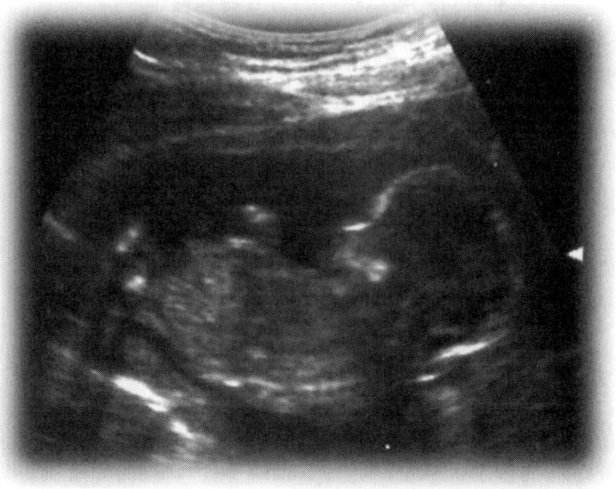

DAY 108

Babies are becoming active and quiet with a degree of regularity or circadian rhythmicity. Continuous ultrasound recording of babies' movements found that the peak of fetal activity occurs in the late evening (8-11 pm) which is consistent with what mothers report. Activity is quietest during the early hours of the day. Circadian rhythms are tied to external events in the environment like light and dark periods, and are controlled by areas in the brain located in the hypothalamus. Interestingly, this late evening peak of activity will be lost immediately after birth.

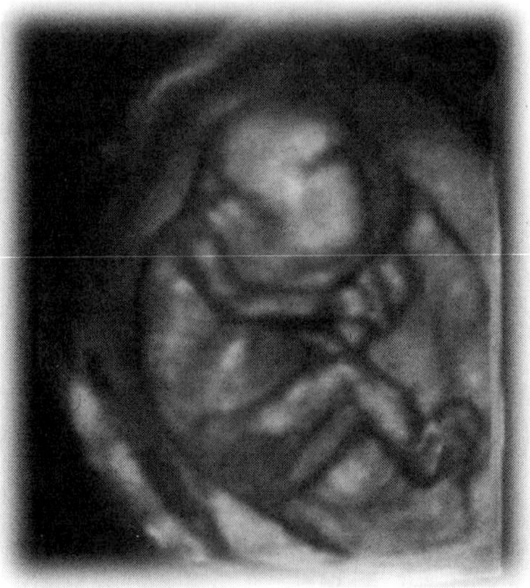

Thoughts:

....

....

DAY 109

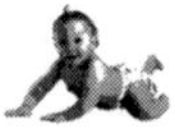

The digestive system, including the stomach, is working. Operating on swallowed amniotic fluid, digestive glands function and the baby generates urine which is released into the amniotic fluid. There are no solid waste products in the developing intestine yet.

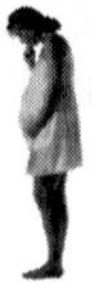

Sleeping on your side may be more comfortable and your baby will receive maximum circulation if you sleep on your left side. Some women find it comfortable to place a pillow between their knees while sleeping.

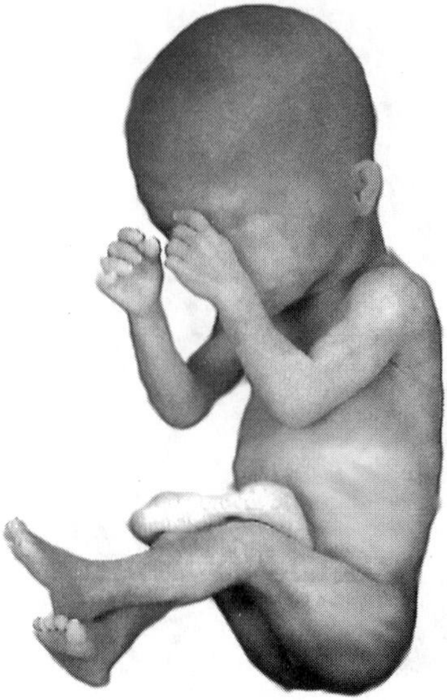

Notes:

....

....

DAY 110

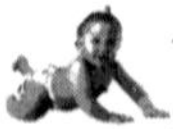

As you can see the baby legs are developed and muscular enough to generate quite a kick. If you haven't felt kicks yet you will soon. Salivary glands are functional.

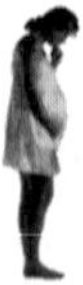

Due to the growth of your uterus and baby, your bladder has become compressed. It now can hold less urine, so you'll have to make more frequent trips to the bathroom.

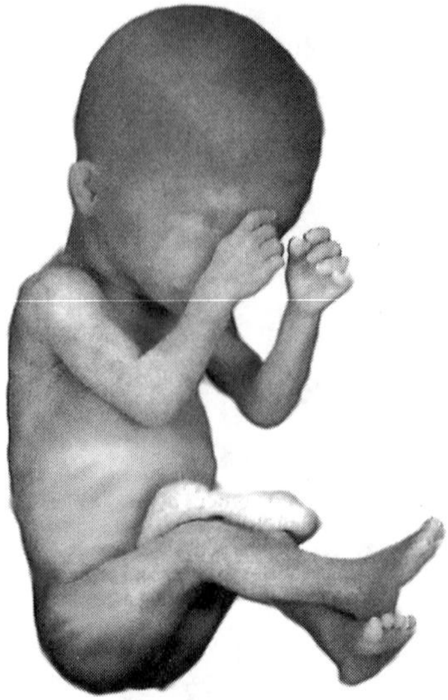

Thoughts:

....

....

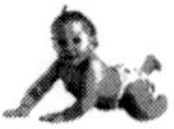

Lots of changes are obviously occurring unseen beneath the skin. Nerve to muscle connections have increased greatly, enabling fine dextrous movements like moving the thumb independently of the fingers. An independent free-moving thumb is essential to fine dextrous movements. The neural real estate in the brain devoted to the thumb is much larger than the other fingers.

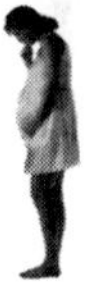

Your heart rate will probably increase somewhat during the course of your pregnancy. Since your blood volume has increased and you've added additional weight in the form of breast, uterine, placental tissues and the baby, your heart will have to work just a little bit harder.

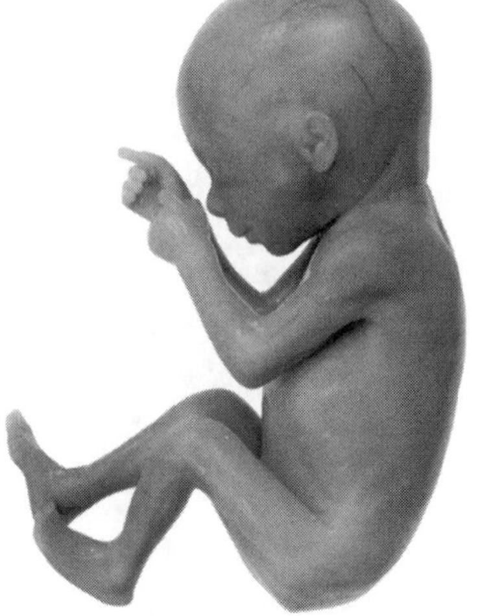

Notes:

....

....

DAY 112

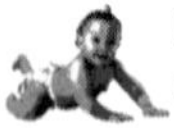

If the sole of the foot is touched, the baby will lift up the stimulated foot and kick out with the other. This reflex resembles the stepping reflex that becomes important around the age of one when your child will be learning to walk.

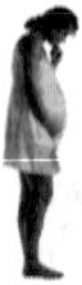

You may notice that a yellowish fluid can be expressed from your breast. This is colostrum; a fluid containing antibodies and protein. Colostrum will nourish your baby for the first few days after birth until your milk comes in. The antibodies also protect your baby from infection by the many germs present in the environment.

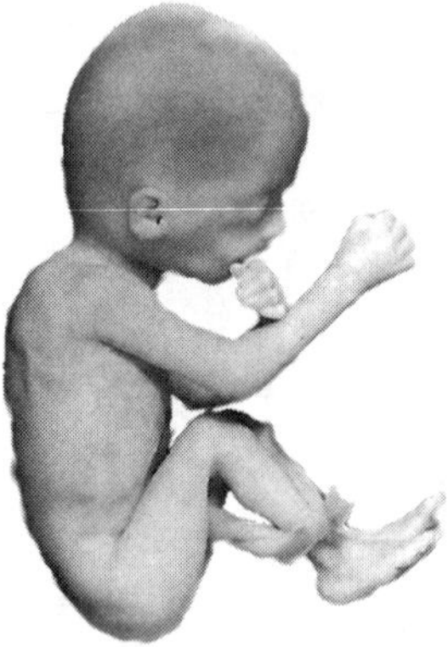

Thoughts:

....

....

DAY 113

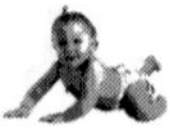

Today begins the 5th month of your pregnancy. The baby is positioned head-up with the legs in the 'fetal' position. And you definitely look pregnant. Your baby will gain about 3 inches in length and about 8 ounces in weight this month to reach a size of about one foot and one pound.

Baby is 9 inches ❦ 8 oz.

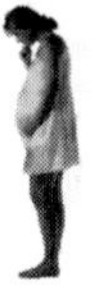

This month's checkup will involve weight and blood pressure measurement, urine sample, fetal heartbeat, measurement of the size and shape of your uterus and a general exam.

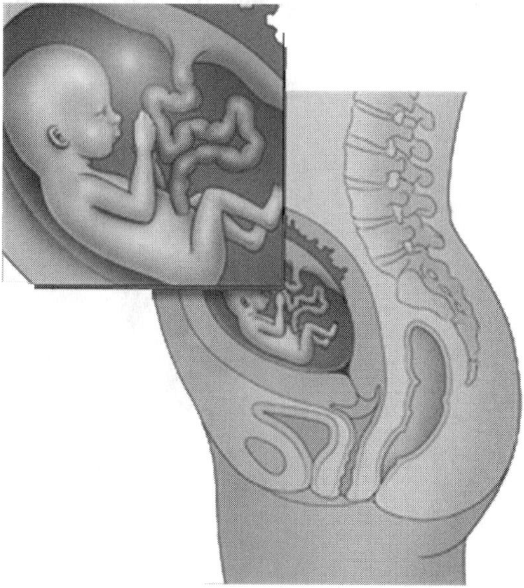

Notes:

....

....

DAY 114

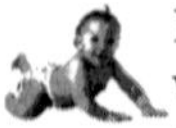

Most babies start moving very early, usually near the 7th week. However, since your baby is so small you probably won't feel anything until now...at the earliest. These movements - known as quickening - will feel like a gentle fluttering sensation. Some women report that the first movements felt are like a butterfly loose inside, or gas bubbles or a ticklish sensation.

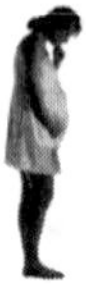

On average, most mothers will usually first feel their baby's movement during this week. First-time mothers usually notice the movement later than more experienced moms who are quicker to recognize the sensation. The average time between when a mother first feels her baby move and birth is 147 days.

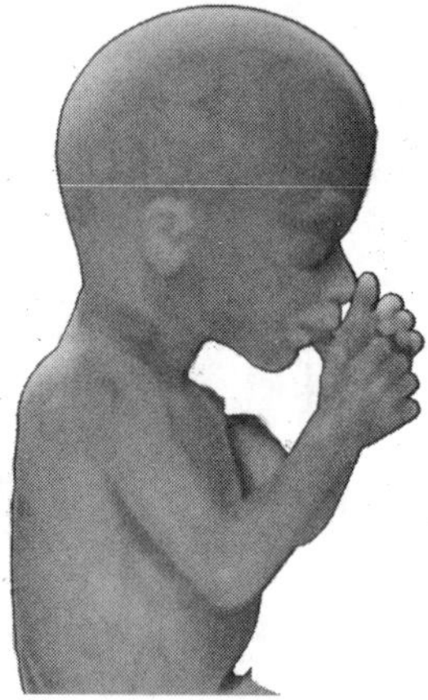

Thoughts:

....

....

DAY 115

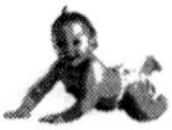

The umbilical cord grows along with your baby. The average length will be about 2 feet. It takes about thirty seconds for substances in the blood to go through the baby's circulation and back through the cord again.

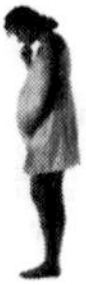

Second-time or more, moms : Most women experience the sensations of expanding and fullness about a month sooner than they did with their first baby. Usually this also means that you felt the baby move about a month earlier than with your first.

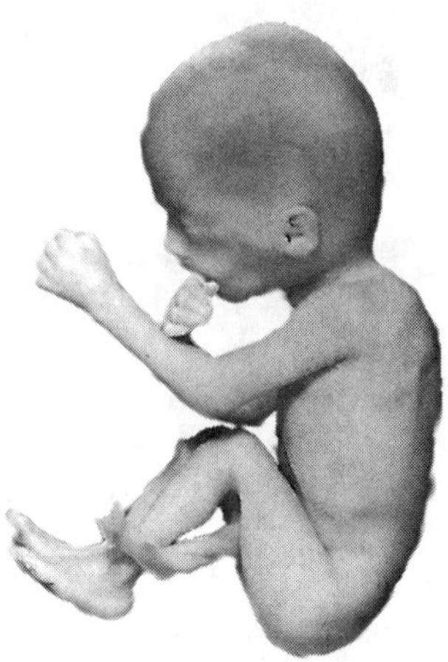

Notes:

....

....

DAY 116

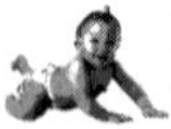

Little, fine hairs known as Laguno hairs are starting to appear on the torso and head. These hairs appear all over the body and disappear by birth. Their function may be to provide surface area or anchoring points for a protective substance that will coat the skin called the vernix caseosa.

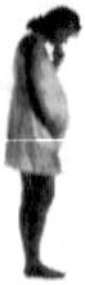

In addition to protein for the growth and development of your baby's tissues, you'll need extra Vitamin A as well. Good sources of Vitamin A are sweet potatoes and carrots.

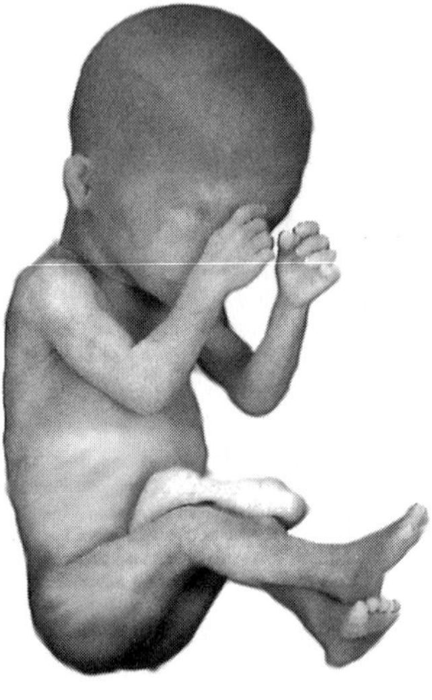

Thoughts:

....

....

DAY 117

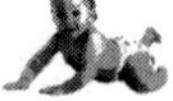

Notice that the baby's ears have moved into their final position. The baby will tug on and pull the umbilical cord, sometimes squeezing hard enough to temporarily slow down the flow of blood. The baby can't hurt itself by pulling on the cord.

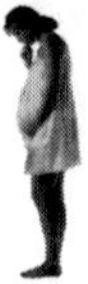

As your skin starts to stretch you may notice more itching. Keeping your skin moistened with a good moisturizer or baby oil will ease the drying and control the itch.

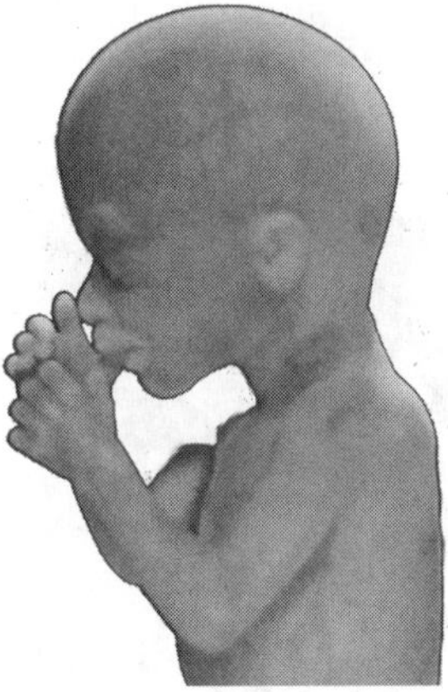

Notes:

....

....

DAY 118

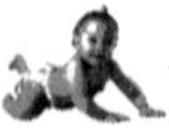

In the next few weeks your baby will double its weight! The baby is getting large enough to occupy most of the space in the uterus...so much so that now the head will be forced down and the legs pulled up to the chest. This is the fetal position.

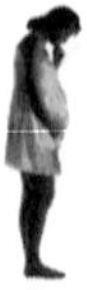

Pregnant women need water. Water helps carry nutrients to your baby via your blood. Water also helps keep your urine diluted, which can help prevent bladder infections. Water can also prevent constipation and hemorrhoids.

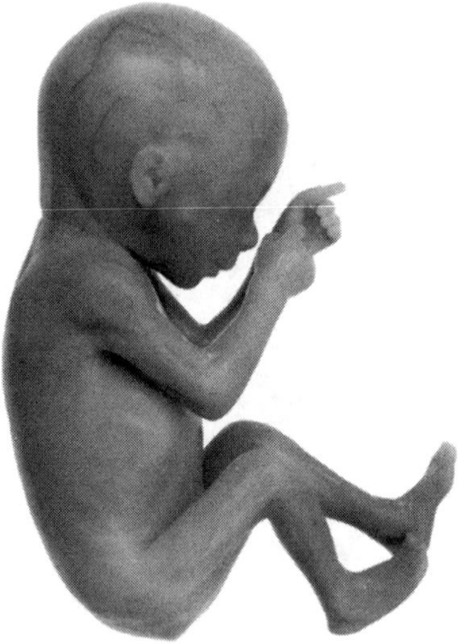

Thoughts:

....

....

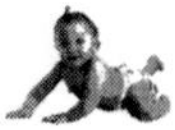

Your baby is most likely positioned upright in your uterus, surrounded by about 350 ml of amniotic fluid. The skin will start to be covered by a substance known as vernix caseosa - a mixture of fatty secretions. This substance protects the baby's delicate skin from scratches and hardening. It is the creamy white coating that you may have seen on photos of newborn babies.

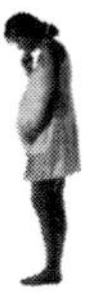

How much water? Drink at least 6-8 eight ounce glasses a day. Coffee, tea and colas don't count because they're diuretics - which cause your body to excrete water.

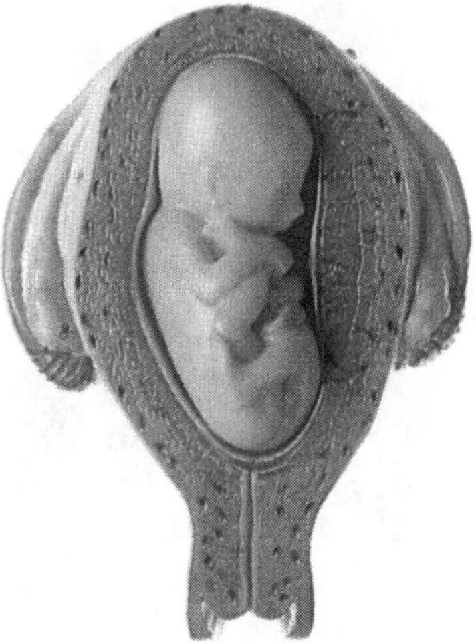

Notes:

DAY 120

The womb is starting to get a little snug. A baby girl will have approximately 2 million eggs in her ovaries which will diminish to about 200,000 by the time she's born. Did you realize that any child has genetic material that is as old as her mother? Your eggs contain your genetic contribution fixed in time when your eggs were formed before you were born.

Baby is 10 inches ❦ 10 oz.

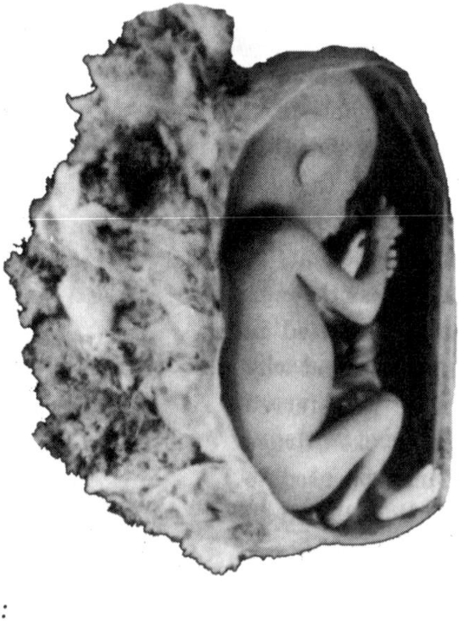

Thoughts:

....

....

DAY 121

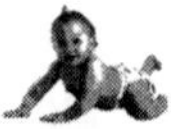

The baby's skeleton is made up of cartilage but many of the bones are calcifying. Particularly, the leg and arms bones will show up as dense objects in an ultrasound scan because they are beginning to harden.

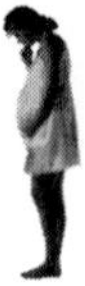

As the baby's bones harden and strengthen the need for calcium is increasing. Drink lots of milk and eat other dairy products. If there is not sufficient extra calcium in your diet the baby will take more calcium from your bones. This could lead to problems down the road like osteoporosis.

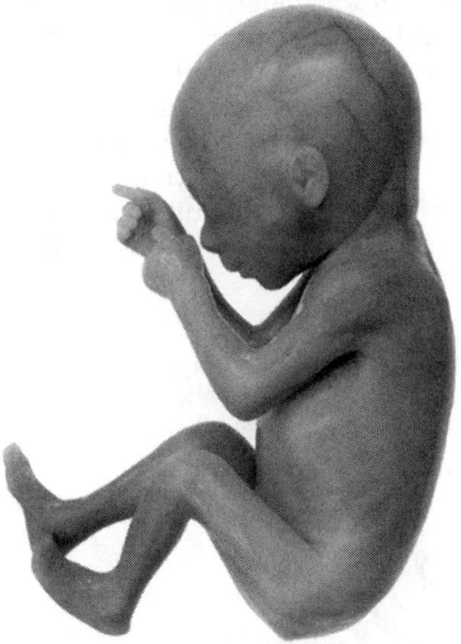

Notes:

....

....

DAY 122

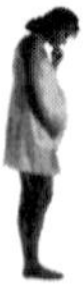

At some point during pregnancy, just about every woman misplaces her keys, forgets why she went to the store, or forgets the name of her pet because her mind is temporarily out to lunch. This frustrating absent mindedness is usually written off to stress or distraction, but here's a new explanation: brain shrinkage. A study has found that pregnant women's brains get smaller in the third trimester. British researchers scanned the brains of ten moms-to-be during their last trimesters and again a few months after their babies were born and made the astounding discovery that brain cell volume decreases during pregnancy, only to plump up again sometime after delivery. The researchers speculate that hormones cause the shrinkage; they hope further study will prove their hypothesis. Another study conducted by a University of Southern California psychologist found that women also suffer from impaired cognitive function while pregnant, with neither their short-term memories nor their concentration and ability to retain new information up to par. What's a mother to do? To retain your sanity, make lists, leave yourself notes, and keep a tight grip on those keys.

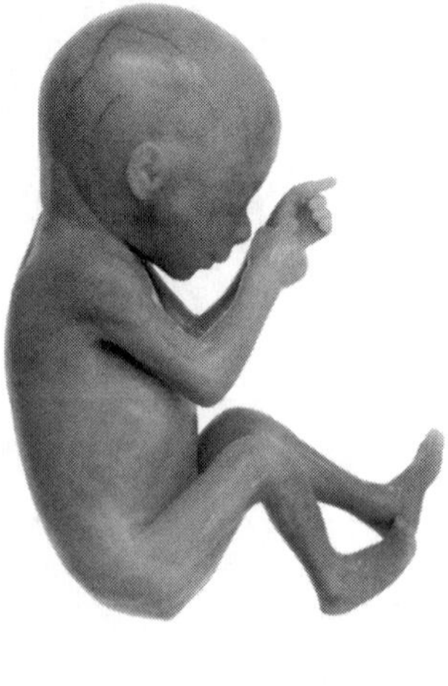

DAY 123

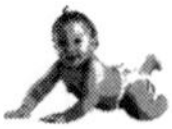

Your baby will have its favorite sleeping position or 'lie.' Remember that the amniotic fluid bath creates an almost weightless environment for the baby to cavort and sleep in. A basic rest and activity cycle is present which will mature into an integrated sleep/wake cycle soon. Your baby can be awakened from sleep by outside noise or bumps. You'll feel increased activity and stirring from your baby when it wakes up.

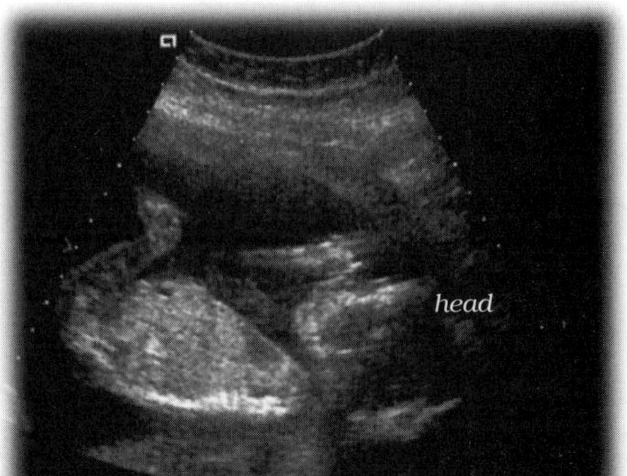

Notes:

....

....

DAY 124

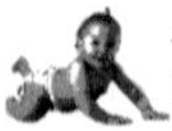

As your baby's bones solidify (or ossify), those kicks and punches will have more umph. You may especially notice a stout kick if your baby is awakened by a loud noise or jolt. This startle response is a complex, integrated response similar to that shown by an adult. Sometimes when the baby is startled it will urinate into the amniotic fluid.

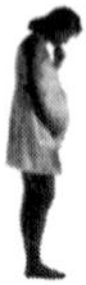

Staying active during your pregnancy has many benefits. Mild exercise usually gives you more energy because it strengthens your cardiovascular system and you don't get tired as easily.

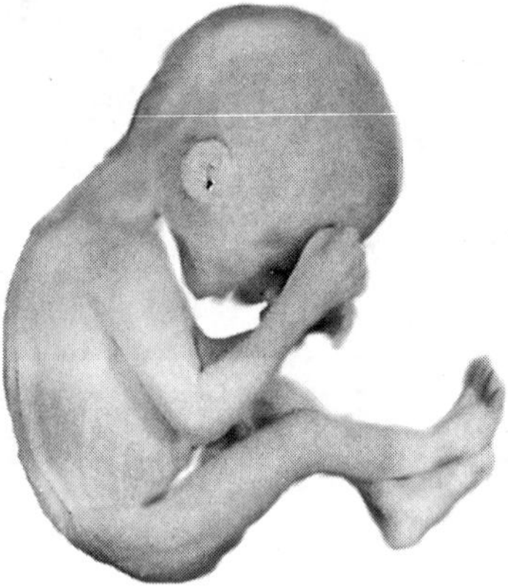

Thoughts:

....

....

DAY 125

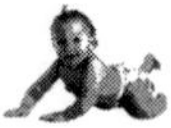

If you look closely, you can see that hair is forming just a little at the top of the head. In a few weeks some babies will have almost a full head of hair. The thyroid gland in the neck is releasing thyroxin - a major hormone involved in regulating metabolism and energy levels.

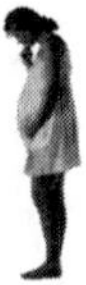

Staying active will help you during delivery by helping maintain your strength and conditioning in the weeks and months leading up to birth. It's called labor because childbirth requires stamina, strength and determination. Plus if you maintain a mild to moderate exercise routine you'll have less distance to travel to get back to your pre-pregnancy form after birth.

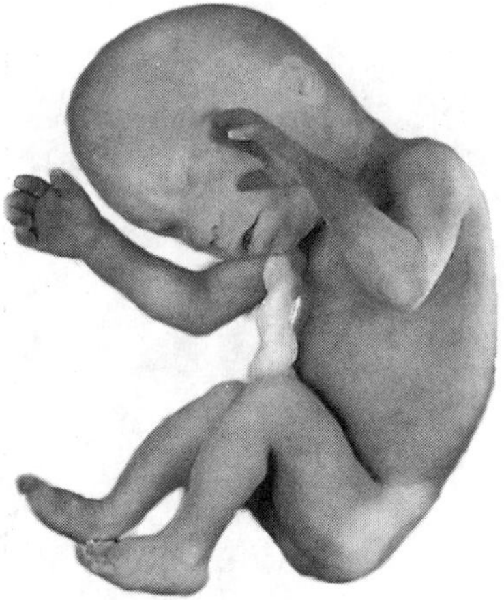

Notes:

....

....

DAY 126

The outer part of the brain - the cortex - is wrinkled and grooved in the adult. Now your baby's cortex is smooth with only the main fissure or space that separates the two halves of the brain clearly defined. The region of the brain devoted to receiving touch information from the hand, and moving the fingers and hand, is relatively large and well-developed.

During pregnancy women are especially prone to urinary tract infections because of changes in the anatomy of the kidneys and bladder. The ducts that run from the kidneys to the bladder can become compressed because of the tight space from the expanding uterus. As a result, incomplete emptying of the bladder can cause infections.

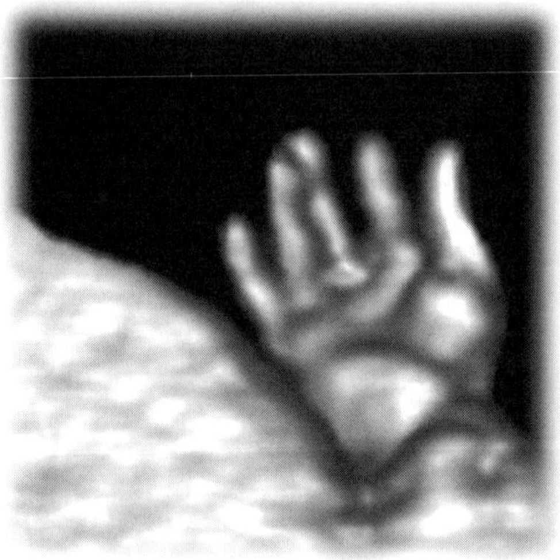

DAY 127

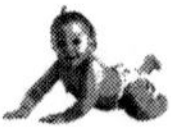

This is about the earliest age from which a premature baby has survived. As you can see in this image, the eyelids are just beginning to separate. Eyebrows start to grow and eyelashes appear on the borders of the fused eyelids. Behind the scenes, the retina, cornea and lens components of the eye are fully formed and waiting for completion of the optic nerve to transmit visual signals to the brain.

Baby is 11 inches ❦ 12 oz.

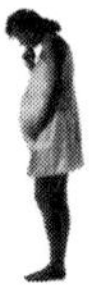

Vitamin D is a fat-soluble vitamin that your body needs for growth, particularly since Vitamin D is important in the utilization of calcium and phosphorus that will make your baby's bones. You can get your daily dose of Vitamin D just by being out in the sun for about 15 minutes per day. Taking a walk will get you your Vitamin D and help you stay active.

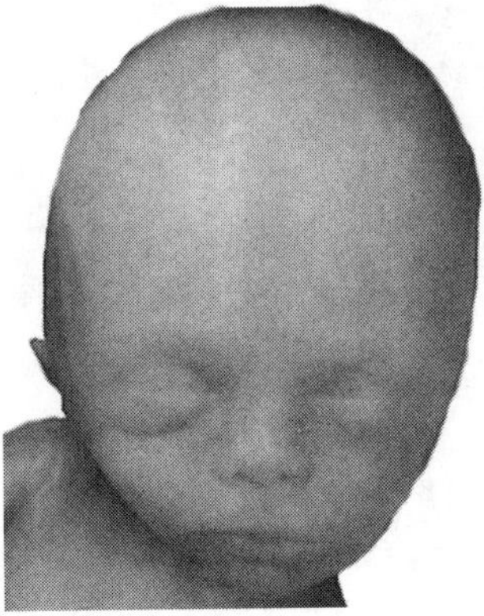

Notes:

....

....

DAY 128

The external ear (pinna) has completed it's development. Did you know that each ear has it's own unique pattern of swirls and curves so intricate that each individual's ear-print is as unique as each fingerprint?

Thiamine (Vitamin B_1) is important for the development of your baby's brain and it helps convert carbohydrates into energy for you. Pork is a great source of thiamine, as are enriched cereals and breads. A woman needs 1.5 mg/day during pregnancy, up from 1.1 mg/day normally.

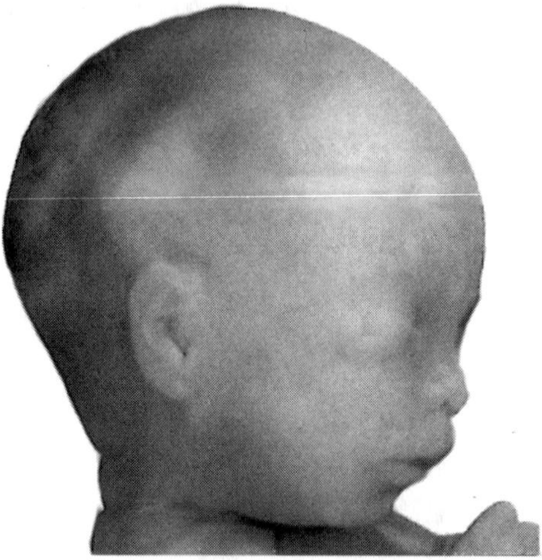

Thoughts:

....

....

The amniotic shell is a silvery white casing with a little over 1 quart of fluid. The amniotic fluid helps keep a constant environment for the fetus, regulating temperature and providing a weightless environment for movement. Suspension in fluid facilitates exercising and development of muscle strength. Floating in the fluid provides few contact or resistance points, facilitating symmetrical growth of the limbs.

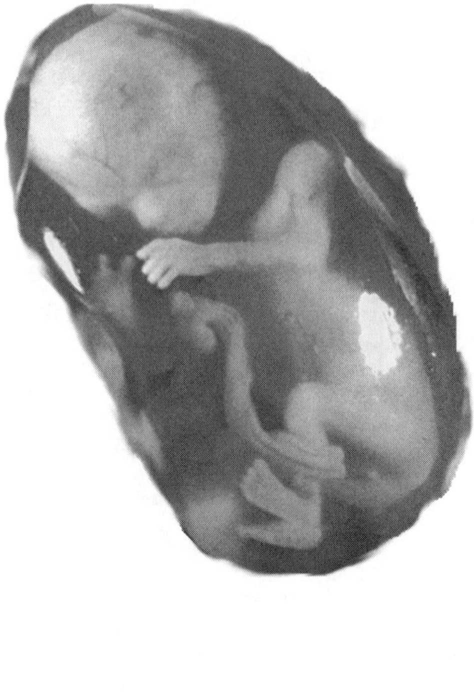

DAY 130

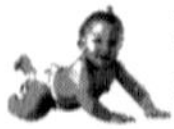

Depending on the position of your baby, the heartbeat is so robust that it may be heard with a simple stethoscope placed on your abdomen. Placing an ear to your abdomen can also enable someone to hear the baby's heart beat.

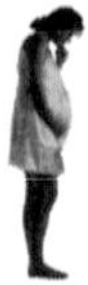

Mild uterine contractions called Braxton Hicks contractions can occur from this point on. These involve tensing and hardening of the uterus for about 30-60 sec. These contractions come and go, and do not mean that you are about to go into labor. Braxton Hicks is just the body's way to warm up to the task of labor that is still many weeks away.

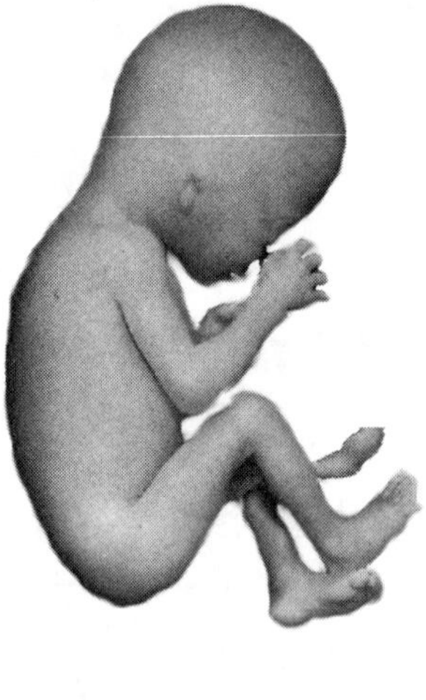

Thoughts:

....

....

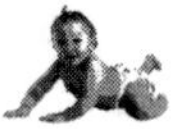

Your baby's movements (kicking, turning, elbowing) may have been felt since the early part of this month (Day 113 or so). They'll get stronger and more noticeable now. You may also feel a rhythmic tapping or light knocking sensation lasting for up to 20-30 minutes...this is your baby hiccuping. Hiccups exercise the intercostal muscles and diaphragm which will help prepare her for when she has to take her first breath of air.

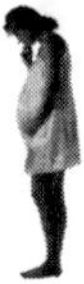

Pregnant women typically need an extra 300 calories per day to support the nutritional demands of the pregnancy. You will probably gain between 12 - 14 lbs. during the second trimester.

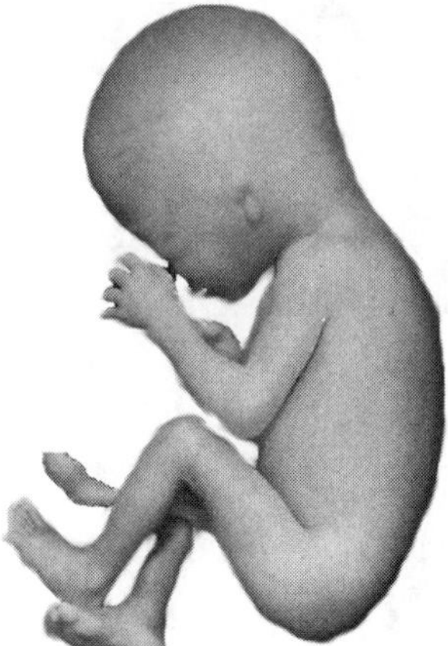

Notes:

....

....

DAY 132

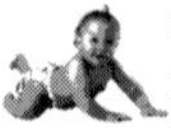

Some of the parts of the brain involved in several types of memory are developed and have been functioning for some time. The nerves responsible for movement have begun to myelinate, which will enhance the fluidity and coordination of movement. Growth hormone is present in the pituitary.

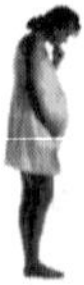

Some herbs that are commonly used in folk or herbal medicine can have adverse effects during pregnancy. Some of the herbs to be avoided are: aloe vera, arbor vitae, clove oil, dong quai, feverfew, juniper oil, mugwort, and sassafras. Most of these, in higher doses, stimulate the uterus to contract, leading to premature labor-like symptoms.

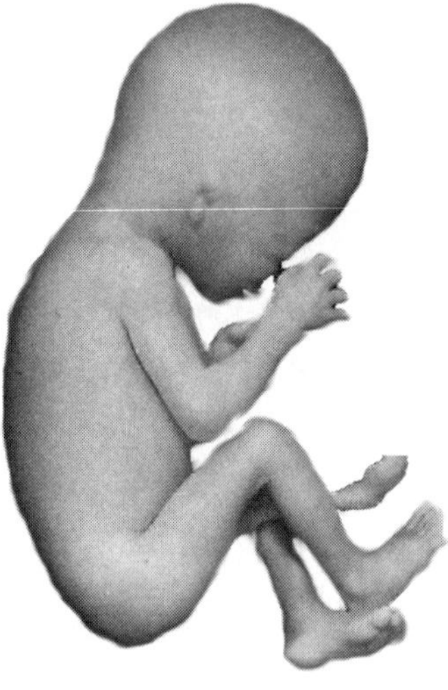

Thoughts:

....

....

DAY 133

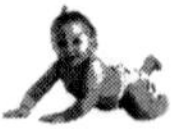

The spinal cord is ossifying in the lower sacral regions, resulting in a straightening of the baby's back and less flexibility compared to earlier periods. The lungs are starting to manufacture a substance called surfactant. This prevents the gas exchange areas of the lungs (the alveloi) from sticking together during respiration. A deficiency in surfactant is a major cause of respiratory distress syndrome in premature babies. New compounds that mimic surfactant can help babies born very early. The lungs will continue to grow by adding alveoli until about 8 years of age.

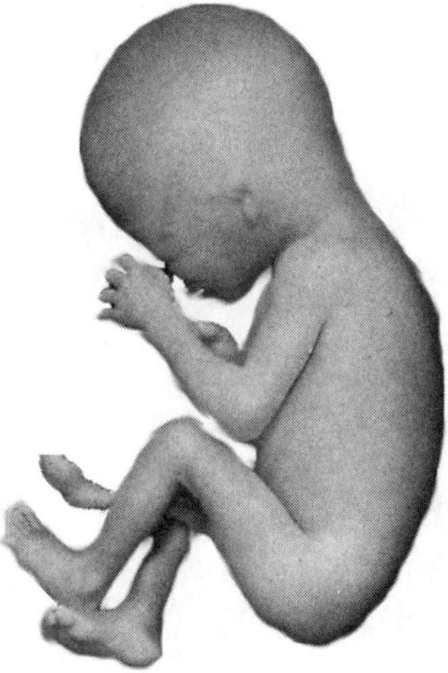

Notes:

....

....

DAY 134

Now, at the latest, the major organ of hearing - the cochlea - is mature and functional. This means that your baby can now hear. What can it hear? All the grumblings of your digestive system, your heart beating and your voice. In fact, compared to external sounds, which are greatly reduced in intensity, your voice is only reduced a negligible amount by the time it passes through the amniotic fluid and reaches your baby's ears. It is learning the intonations of your spoken language and will incorporate some of this learning into the sounds embedded in its cries.

Baby is 12 inches ❦ 12-1/2 oz.

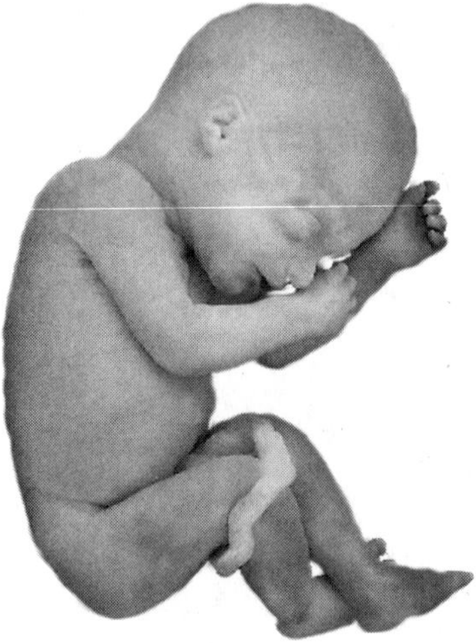

Thoughts:

....

....

DAY 135

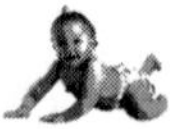

Nails start to grow on the fingers and will extend to the fingertip by the 8th month. When your baby is born, chances are her nails will need to be trimmed. The baby starts to put on weight by laying down layers of fat. The areas of the brain involved in processing the outside world are maturing.

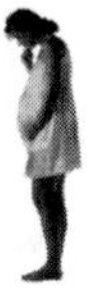

The surge in progesterone causes you to dream more frequently and those dreams can be more dramatic and more vivid. Dreams incorporate the happenings of waking life into their content. Since the baby and the prospect of motherhood is coming it is normal that your dreams reflect these impending changes.

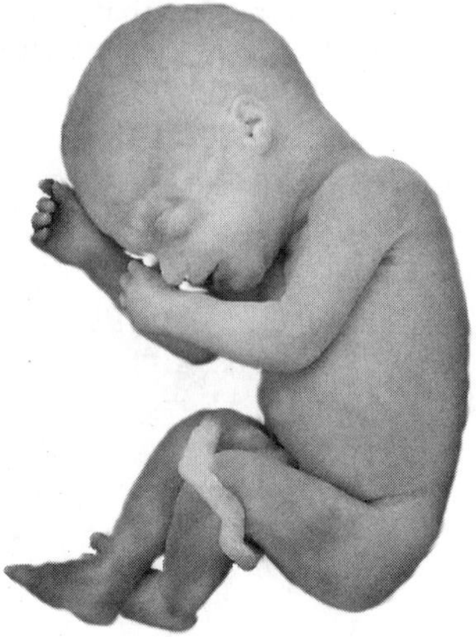

Notes:

....

....

DAY 136

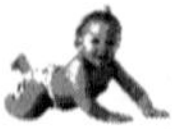

Brain cells operate by releasing chemicals (neurotransmitters) to influence the activity of other neurons. Some neurotransmitters have been shown to operate differently before birth than they do later. For example GABA, a key neurotransmitter in the brain, blocks or inhibits the activity of neurons in the mature brain. But in the fetal brain it has the exact opposite effect - it makes the neuron more active. So there is evidence of a radical difference in the operation of the brain in the fetus compared to the child or adult.

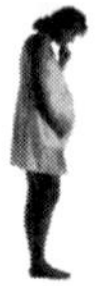

There is a consensus of evidence that women who smoke while breastfeeding nurse their babies for a shorter duration. However, the search for a physiological cause has not be fruitful. Some studies suggest that smoking (nicotine) inhibits oxytocin release which would interfere with the milk let down reflex. However, this finding is not conclusive.

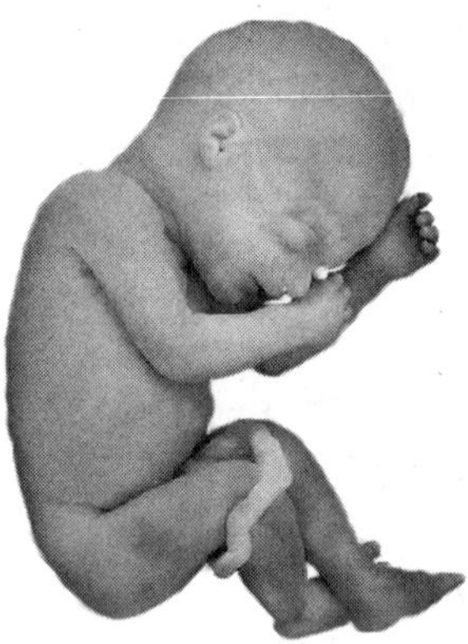

Thoughts:

....

....

DAY 137

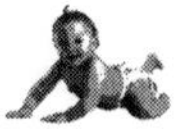

Your baby's grip is very strong - with the baby capable of lifting itself by the strength of its grip in certain experimental settings. Some theorize that this grip is an evolutionary leftover trait enabling furry ape infants to grasp their mother's fur to facilitate suckling, transport and protection.

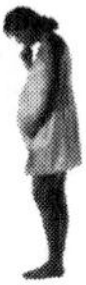

Depression during pregnancy affects about 10% of all pregnant women. Between hormonal changes, fatigue and the imminent personal and financial changes, a higher level of stress can be experienced.

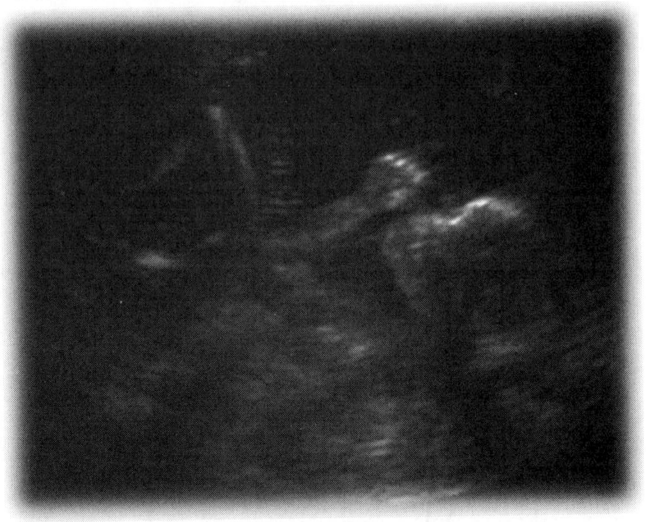

Ultrasound image of baby sucking thumb

DAY 138

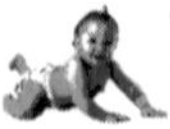

Your baby's hands are shown at rest (A) and following a light touch of the palm (B). At rest the palm is exposed and the fingers including the thumb are partially bent - similar to how an adult hand appears at rest. When touched in the palm a grasp reflex is elicited in which the fingers close around the object, as if to grasp it. Now all fingers are involved and the thumb closes as well. This is a mature grasp reflex.

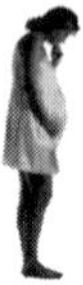

Depression is distinctly different from the moodiness that can accompany pregnancy. Inability to concentrate, anxiety, extreme irritability, constant fatigue, persistent sadness, sleep problems, change in eating habits (eating all the time or no desire to eat) and a sense that nothing is fun or enjoyable anymore are signs to watch out for with depression. If you experience any or some of these symptoms let your doctor know.

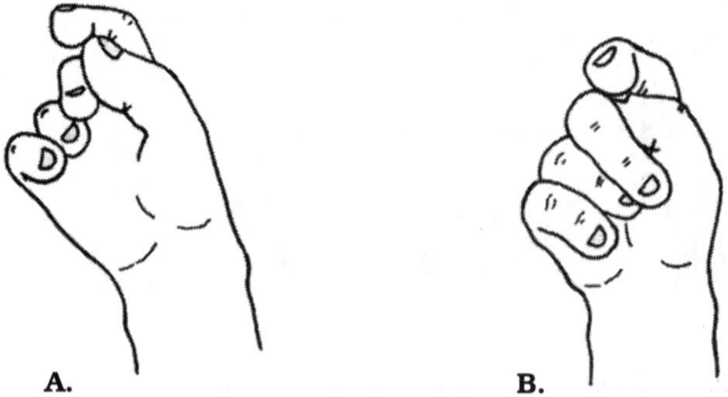

A. **B.**

from Humphrey (1964).

DAY 139

Your baby is constantly swallowing and processing tastes in the amniotic fluid. An interesting study has shown that newborns react with a 'surprise' reaction to tastes like sweet, sour, and bitter but not to salty tastes. This shows that since salt is the predominant taste of amniotic fluid, the baby *remembers* the familiar taste from her days as a fetus. Remember how other studies have shown that babies prefer sweet over sour substances injected into the amniotic fluid way back at 12 weeks? Think about what these results may mean - discriminating between tastes may indicate the presence of early emotional states (pleasure, displeasure) and the learning and retention of basic taste information acquired early on in development.

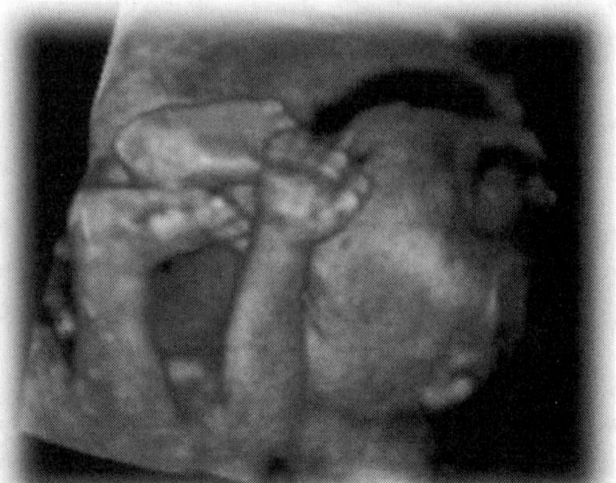

Notes:

....

....

DAY 140

Your baby is about halfway through the gestational period. Movements have become more complex involving the hips, elbows and trunk. Movement will help sculpt the structure of the developing joints and define the range of movement of the limbs.

The temporary changes in your body may have made you a little more clumsy that usual. The enlarged torso, loosening of your pelvic joints and the center of gravity shifts that resemble a gyroscope movement when the baby shifts position, all contribute to upsetting your usual balance and grace.

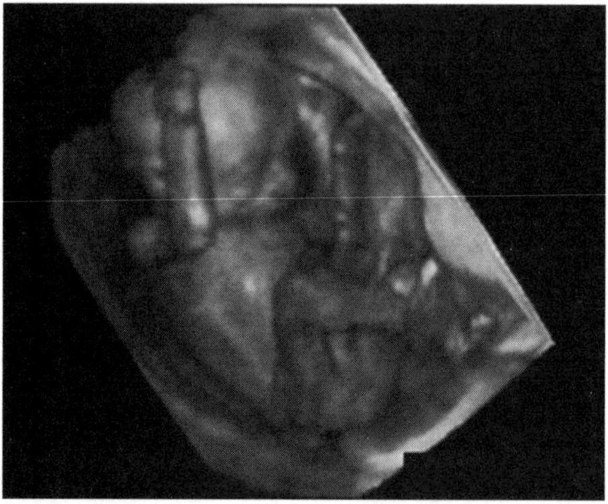

Thoughts:

....

....

DAY 141

Since the 16th week the weight of the baby has doubled to about 15 ounces, length is about 12 inches.

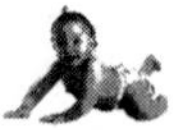

This is the time to start looking into childbirth classes and preparing for the details of the birth. Stay active and maintain good nutritional habits. This month's checkup will involve weight and blood pressure measurement, urine sample, fetal heartbeat, fetal size, measurement of the size and shape of your uterus and a general exam.

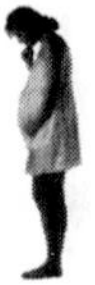

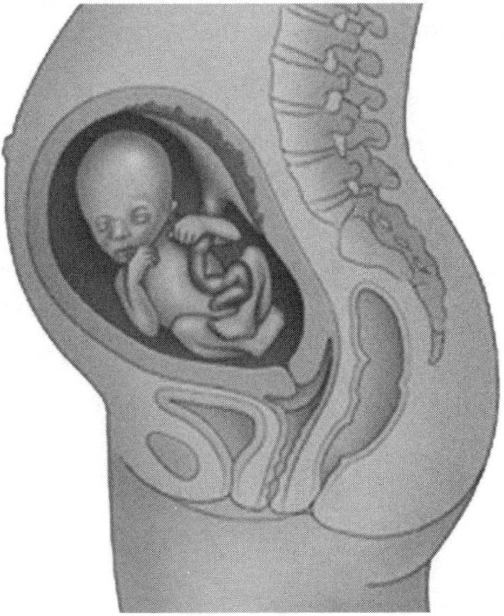

Notes:

....

....

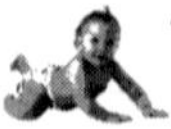

The testes of a boy baby will start their descent into the scrotum now. Ovaries will remain in place. Rapid eye movements occur now in addition to slow, smooth eye movements.

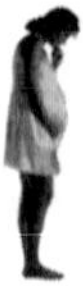

Pregnant beauty - People will tell you how beautiful you are, even though you may have difficulty accepting the changes pregnancy has had on your body. Your skin, hair and overall appearance has changed. A pregnant woman is always noticed. People may be responding to the thrill of a new life and sharing in the excitement you are feeling. Enjoy center stage attention now - your new baby will be the show stopper in a few months.

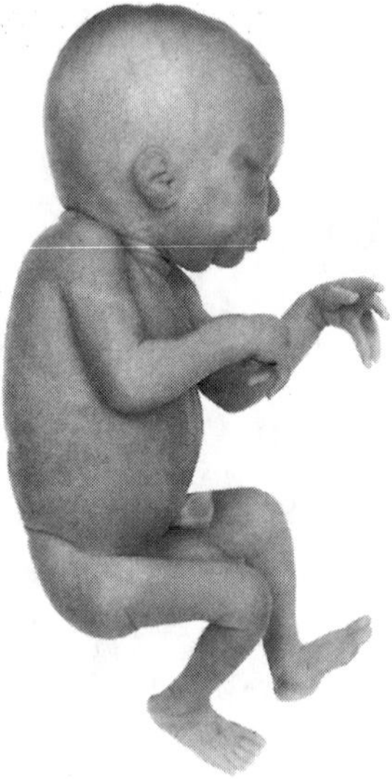

Thoughts:

....

....

DAY 143

Brown fat cells, which are heat-producing, are deposited in the neck and chest region as well as the groin area. This gives the baby a chubby look. These brown fat stores will disappear by birth, replaced with white fat cells distributed under the skin.

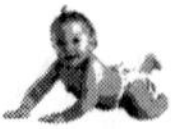

The need for calcium is greatest from here on out because the baby's skeleton is rapidly ossifying or hardening. About 13 mg of calcium per hour pass through the placenta into the baby now. Calcium is best utilized if it is taken in natural forms such as in milk, cheese or yogurt.

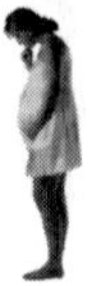

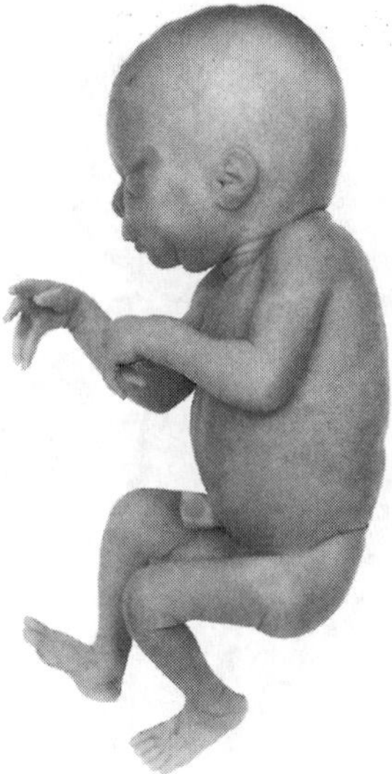

Notes:

....

....

DAY 144

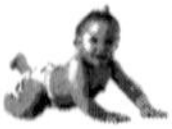

By 6 months, all the components of the auditory system are structurally complete and have mature microscopic characteristics. In other words, the baby has all the apparatus to hear.

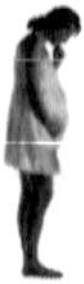

Maintaining good postural habits will enhance your comfort as you get larger. Stand with your head held high and chin level; this will help align the rest of your body. Have your shoulders back and relaxed, abdominal muscles firm and your back slightly curved inward. Poor posture can cause backaches because your muscles must work harder to maintain proper body alignment and balance.

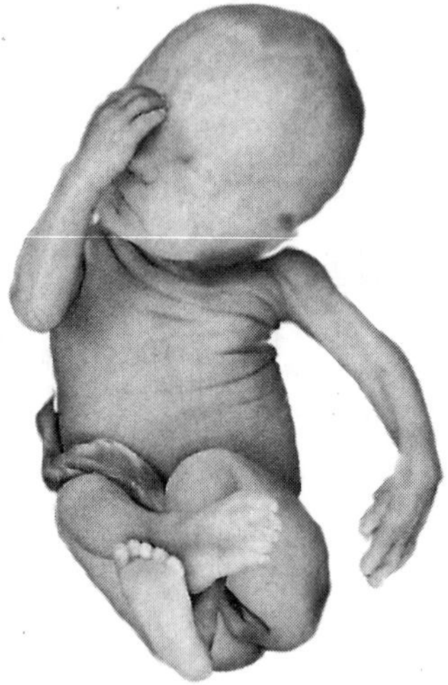

Thoughts:

....

....

DAY 145

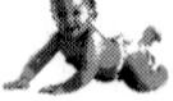

Intrauterine temperature is a steady 1.0 - 2.7 degrees F above that of the mother. The baby can not thermoregulate (control its own body temperature) yet but the amniotic fluid keeps the baby warm and cozy.

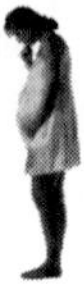

Use common sense to maintain your comfort. Wear low-heeled or flat shoes or sneakers; comfortable loose-fitting clothing that won't constrict or restrict movement. When standing, don't stand in one place too long. Alternately shift your weight from one leg to another to keep blood moving and to distribute the work around your body.

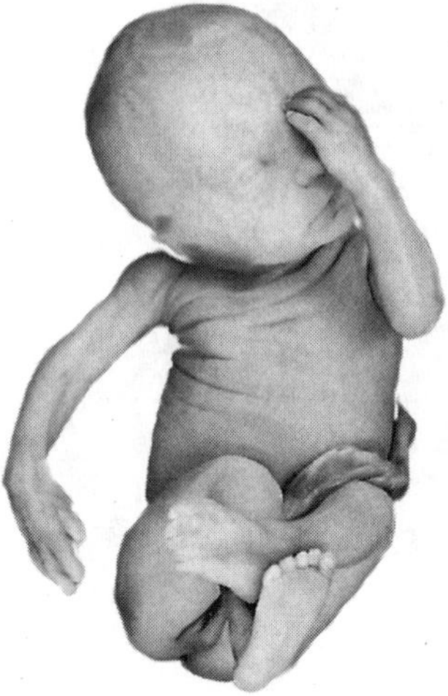

Notes:

....

....

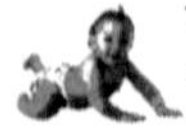

What is your baby tasting? Amniotic fluid is always changing in amount and the substances suspended in it -- some 390 substances have been identified. Glucose, fructose; lactic, pyruvic and citric acids; fatty acids; phospholipids; creatine; urea; uric acid; amino acids; proteins and salts are some of the tasty substances identified in amniotic fluid. Furthermore, doctors have found that some tasty substances that the mother consumes like curry and garlic will tint the smell and taste of amniotic fluid - what you eat sometimes the baby tastes! So the gustatory environment of your baby is very rich and stimulating.

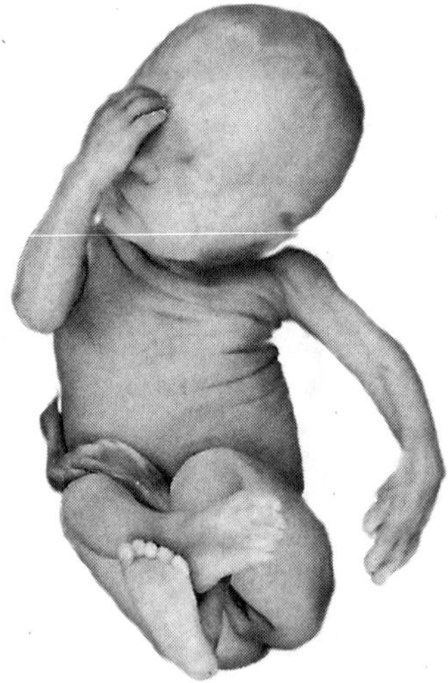

Thoughts:

....

....

DAY 147

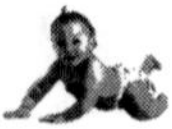

Here is what your baby might look like positioned horizontally in your uterus. It is bathed in about 380 ml (13 fl. oz.) of amniotic fluid. It can pucker its lips as if kissing, and engage in intricate lip protrusion movements too.

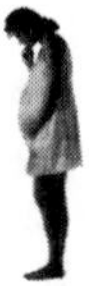

The physical changes in your body make it risky to lift heavy objects now. You can safely lift lighter objects like laundry baskets and groceries only if you pay attention to your posture. Always use your legs, not your back, to lift. Bend at the knees, not the waist. Get near the object, squat down, grab it, draw it near and rise using your legs.

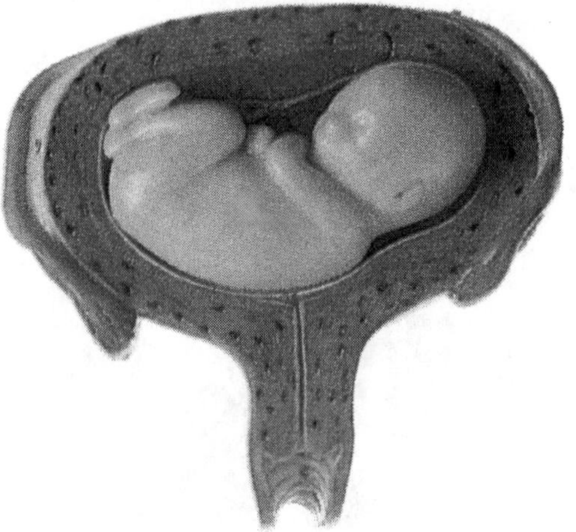

Notes:

....

....

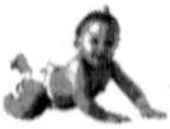

If your were able to see your baby outside the womb its skin would appear very wrinkled and red. The red coloration is because blood in the capillaries in the skin can be seen through the translucent skin.

Baby is 12-1/2 inches ❦ 15 oz.

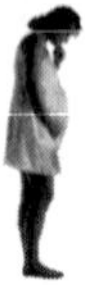

When sitting , get up to move around frequently. Don't cross your legs at the knees as it will cut off circulation. Sit in a firm-back chair (you'll be able to more easily get out of it) with your feet elevated on a stool or ottoman. To avoid straining your back, get up from the chair by first moving to the edge of the seat, use your legs to stand, and push up with your arms as well.

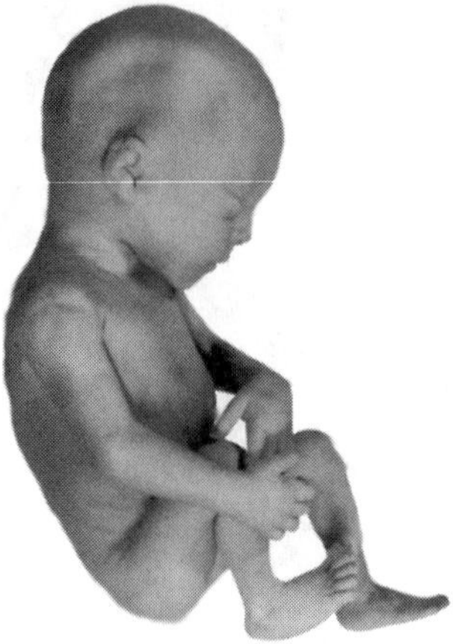

Thoughts:

....

....

DAY 149

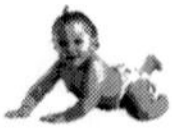

The external surface of the brain (the cortex) has the six distinct layers that are present in adults. Initially, the cortex is smooth. Over the next few weeks the surface of the brain will start to wrinkle and fold in an effort to more efficiently pack more neurons into the confines of the skull.

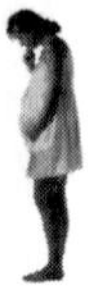

Sitting in a car can be safe and comfortable. Fasten the seatbeat low across your pelvis, under the baby. On long trips, stop when you feel restless and walk around. Get out of the car slowly by pulling yourself up while using your legs. Avoid sudden abrupt movements, because the weight of the baby will lag behind the movement and you will stretch the uterine ligaments.

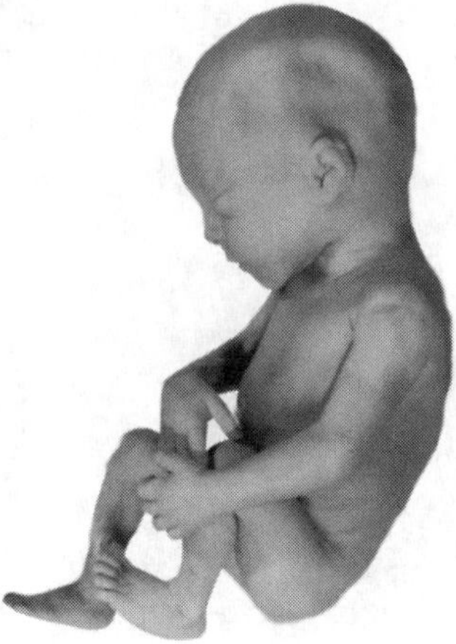

Notes:

....

....

DAY 150

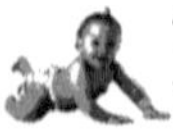

The part of the retina (the fovea) where light is focused develops now. The nerves that relay visual signals to the brain (the optic nerves) are myelinating, which will enable fast clear signal transmission from the retina to the brain.

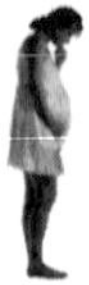

You can't just pop up out of bed now. Get up by first rolling on your side, slowly place your legs over the side of the bed, push yourself up to a sitting position and use your leg muscles to stand. Moving too fast will stretch your uterine ligaments and you'll feel a sharp pain.

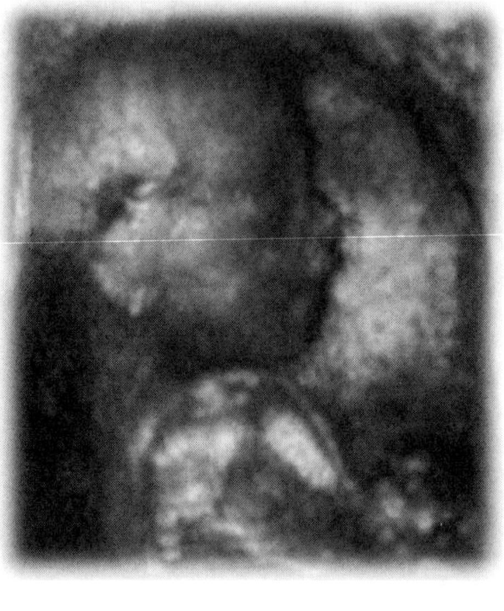

Thoughts:

....

....

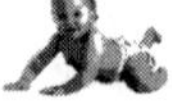

Tear ducts develop, as do other glands that will help bathe and protect the eyes during the lifetime of your child. Crying will be without tears until a few months after birth when the ducts carry fluid. The eyelids are still shut, however, there is lots of eye movement behind the lids. Particularly side-to-side eye movements and your baby can roll her eyes around as well.

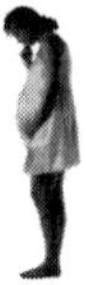

As the baby gets larger you may notice increasing shortness of breath. The expansion capability of your lungs is cramped, so listen to your body and take it easy.

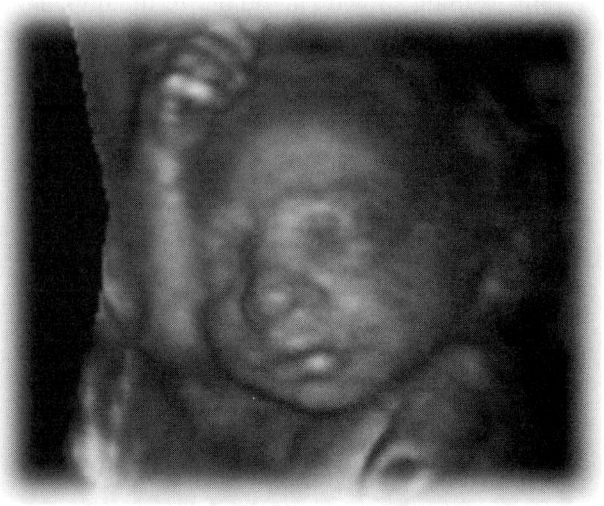

DAY 152

Your placenta is a remarkable organ. It serves as the interface between you and your baby providing a means for your body to nourish the baby and to take away waste products from your baby. The placenta creates many of the hormones that sustain the pregnancy, for example progesterone. Your placenta is a living structure; it consumes about one-third of the oxygen and glucose that passes through it. It is also relatively large - the surface area of the placenta, if unfolded, covers about 900 sq. ft. (that's the floor space of a small condo!)

Some women feel warm or hot during pregnancy regardless of the outside temperature. Since your basal metabolic rate has increased 20%, so you're burning up more calories and generating more heat. Your thermostat is turned up, so layer your clothing so you can adjust to the outside temperature as much as possible.

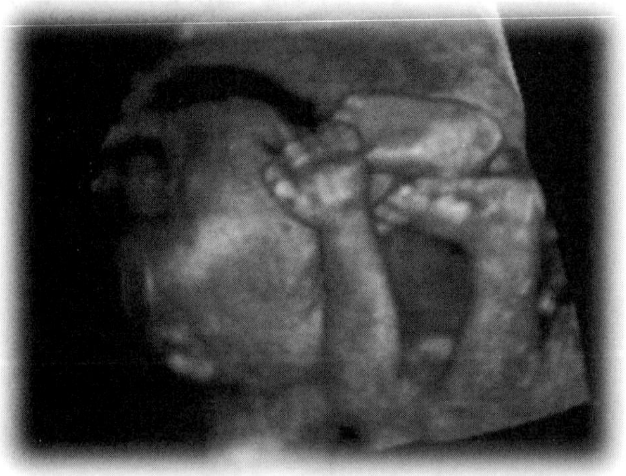

DAY 153

Integrated and coordinated sucking reflexes can be observed now. These involve pursing of the lips and positioning the tongue to enable fluid passage as is seen during normal suckling. Swallowing reflexes have been present for over 10 weeks.

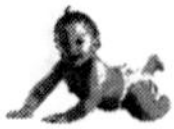

During the course of your pregnancy not only has your body become more efficient at metabolizing and utilizing nutrients, but lung efficiency has increased as well. Your lungs obtained up to 20% more oxygen per breath by Week 20 than they did pre-pregnancy.

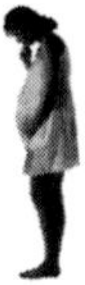

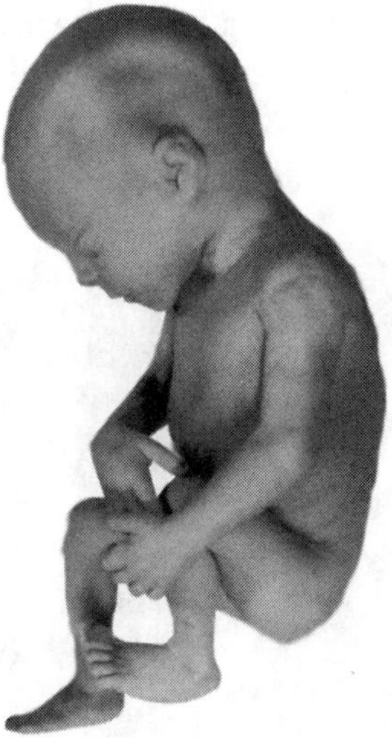

Notes:

....

....

Behavioral responses to sound are present now. Blink and startle responses occur following loud noises outside your abdomen. You may even feel these sudden movements. In response to a loud sound (like dropping a pot lid) your baby will respond with a startle response. This response involves a fast generalized contraction of major muscle groups - legs, arms, trunk. Also there will be an increase in the baby's heart rate following a loud sound. Interestingly, less intense sounds like a phone ringing, will cause the baby's heart rate to decelerate or drop a little. Keep repeating the sound and the heart rate changes decrease. These heart rate responses are important because they show that the baby can hear, and since they decrease over repeated presentations of the sound, demonstrate a very complex form of learning called 'habituation'. Habituation is basically the ability to separate what is new from that which is known...this type of learning occurs in all animals.

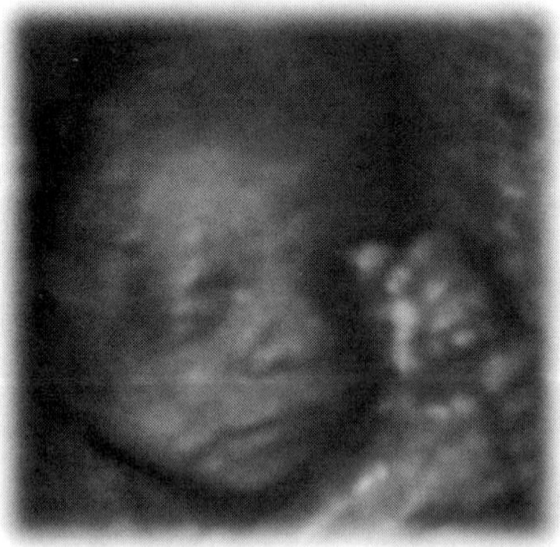

DAY 155

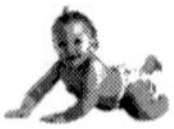

Habituation is viewed as a basic form of learning, perhaps the most important because it essentially helps us separate that which is known from that which is new or novel. When your baby hears a new sound it 'pays attention' and processes the sound and presumably stores a representation of the sound in memory. The measurable evidence of this process is the change in heart rate. Heart rate initially slows down in response to a new sound. Repeat the sound and the heart doesn't decelerate as much. Eventually no heart rate change occurs. What's happening? The baby initially orients to the new sound, learns about it, and puts it in memory. When the sound is heard again, it is recognized as not new and no orienting response (heart rate change) occurs as evidence of that learning. Amazing!

Baby is 13-1/2 inches ❦ 1-1/4 lbs.

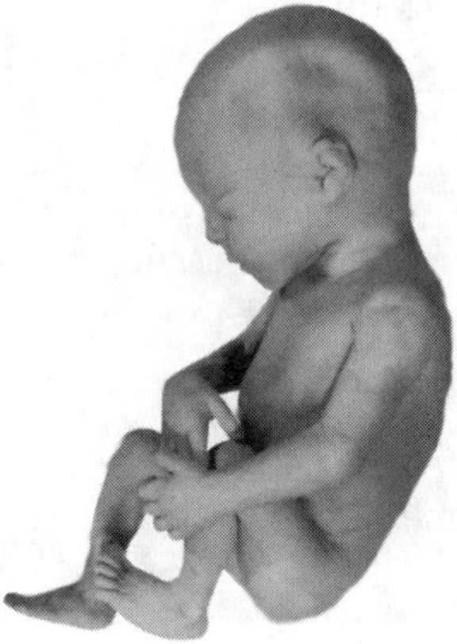

Notes:

....

....

The enamel on the baby teeth of your baby's molars starts to harden. Observations of ultrasound images have shown that after you eat your baby will show increased breathing movements. The functional significance of this relationship is unknown, however, it could simply be related to an increased level of circulating glucose in the blood after your meal. Increased glucose would produce a burst of energy for the baby.

There is some controversy as to whether microwave ovens are a risk to developing babies. Be safe rather than sorry. Don't stand in front of the microwave while it's running and if you're not sure if your oven leaks simple test kits are available at most hardware stores.

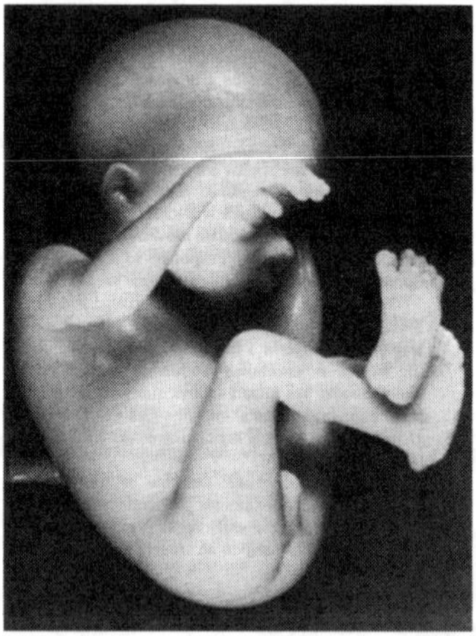

Thoughts:

....

....

DAY 157

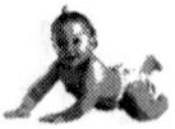

Now that your baby can hear your conversations you'll have to watch what you say. Do babies remember anything from this fetal period? Some studies say yes. One way researchers determine babies' preferences is by measuring their sucking behavior. Babies suck more during preferred and/or familiar stimuli. Studies have shown that newborn babies will suck more when read a story that was repeatedly read to them *in utero* compared to an unfamiliar story...the inference is that they remember the story!

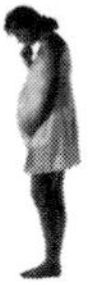

About 96% of all babies are positioned in the head-down or vertex position at birth. 4% are positioned in the head up or breech position.

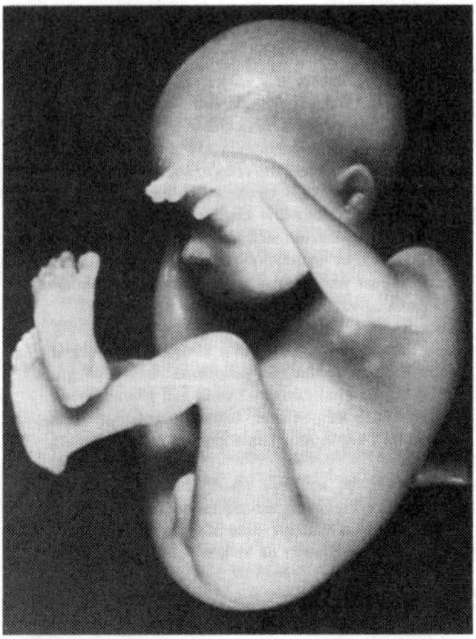

Notes:

....

....

DAY 158

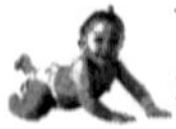

Your baby's brain is buzzing along, but not quite like a newborn's. Recordings of the general neural activity can be obtained as an electroencephalogram (EEG). An EEG is simply a measurement of the general activity of millions of neurons underneath the recording site (usually a spot on the scalp over the frontal cortex). Shown below is a sample of EEG recordings from a baby 23 weeks old. These recordings show slow wave activity indicative of a non-aroused state (although the baby was awake); compared to very fast activity associated with alert wakefulness in the newborn. An important difference can also be that the eyes are open in the newborn but not in the 23 wk old.

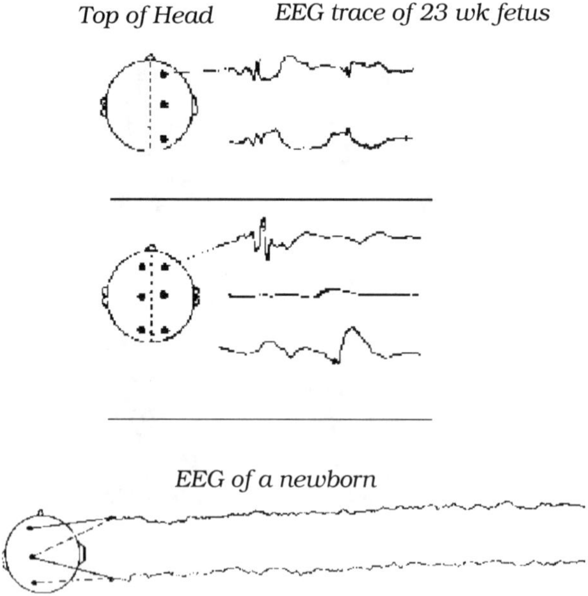

from Sokol & Rosen (1974)

DAY 159

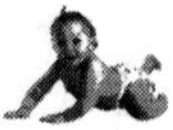

All behavior has an anatomical basis. The EEG tracings taken from the cortex contain neurons like those shown below. The changes that occur in these cells over time contribute to the changes recorded in the EEG. In the top diagram you can see how the neurons grow more complex, with more branches, as your baby gets older. In the bottom diagram you can see the increased complexity of the signal receiving areas of these cells as your baby get older.

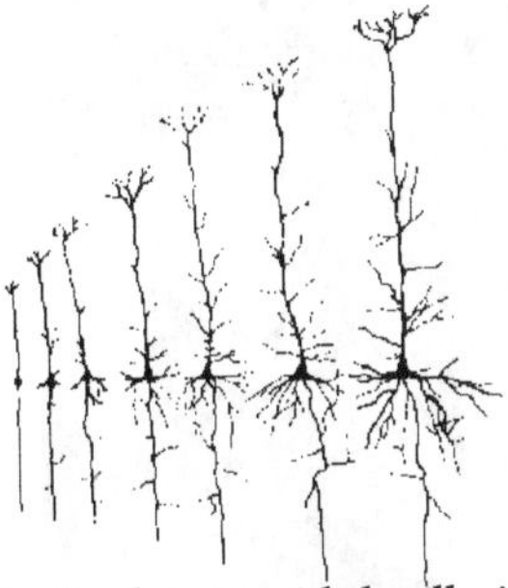

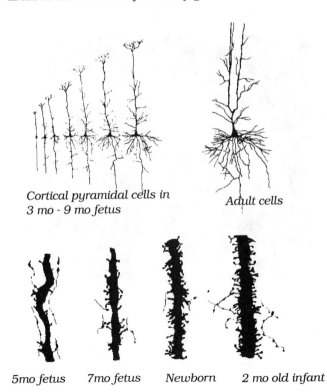

Cortical pyramidal cells in 3 mo - 9 mo fetus

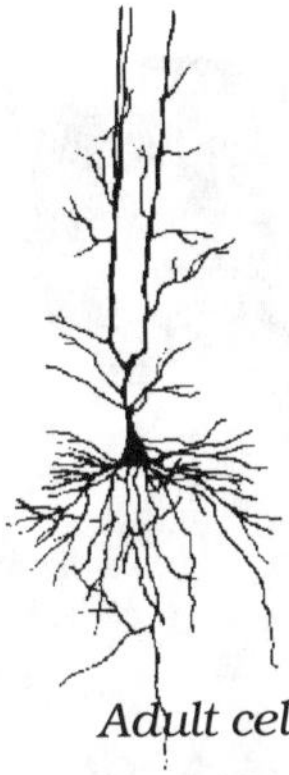

Adult cells

5mo fetus *7mo fetus* *Newborn* *2 mo old infant*

DAY 160

Sleep is changing for your baby with the appearance of rapid eye movement (REM) sleep. REM sleep is also called active sleep because the autonomic nervous system is aroused. Heart rate, blood pressure, breathing movements all increase. The eyes move and the brain is very active. If your baby is a boy he will experience erections like all males do during REM sleep. REM sleep is also the time when we dream. What can your baby be dreaming about?

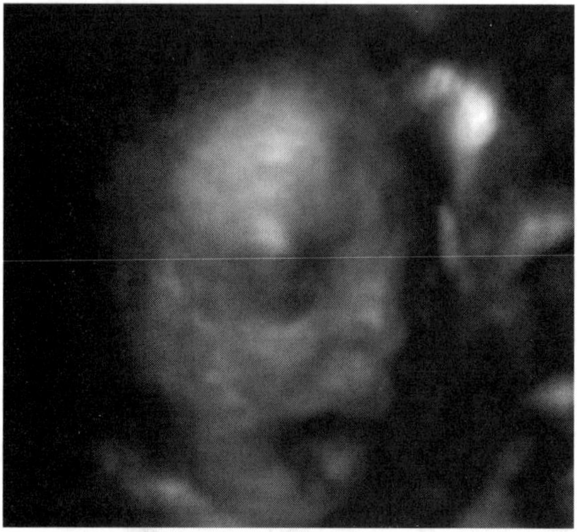

Yawning baby

Thoughts:

....

....

DAY 161

Your baby will spend about 80% of the time it's asleep in REM sleep. This percentage will decrease with age (adults are in REM sleep about 25% of the time). Some scientists think REM sleep exercises the brain and leads to the development of more efficient neural connections. Do you think that your dreams - with its strange sensations like floating and the altered passage of time, etc. - are similar to what you may have experienced when you were in the womb? Some believe that our dreams are a window into the fetal experience - a left over that reminds us where we came from.

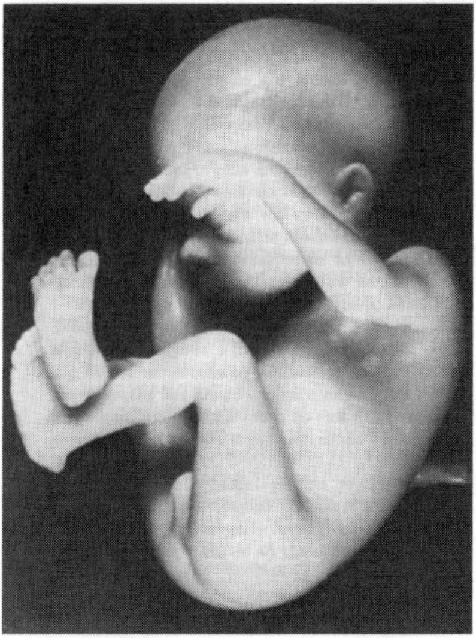

Notes:

....

....

DAY 162

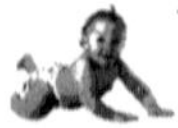

What could your baby be dreaming about? Usually adults incorporate happenings of the day into the content of their nightly dreams. Adults' dreams are also highly visual. Your baby's visual system is probably not adding much input because the eyes are still shut and the uterine space is dark. Interestingly, blind adults do dream and their dreams are composed primarily of sounds. So your child could be incorporating sounds, textures and tastes into the stuff of their dreams.

Baby is 14 inches ❦ 1-1/2 lbs.

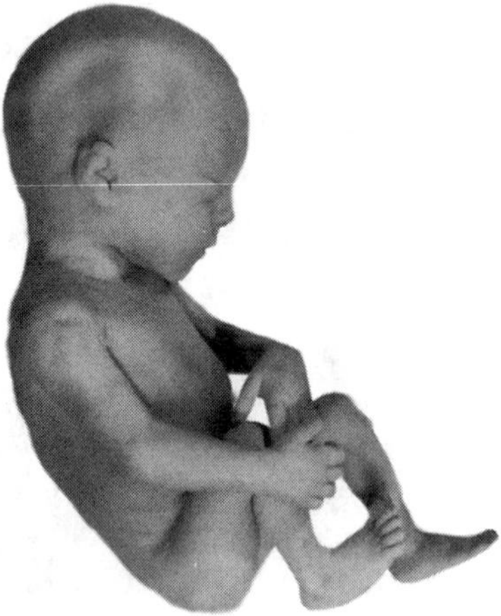

Thoughts:

....

....

DAY 163

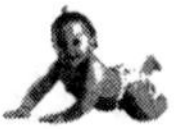

There is an progressive increase in muscle tone (legs and arms pulled up and held for long periods) compared to earlier stages. This is due to the maturation of the cerebellum, a part of the brain that maintains muscle tone. It also facilitates coordination of muscles and is involved in other interesting behaviors.

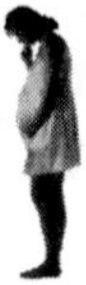

Your breasts will start to feel more lumpy as the milk nodules grow and expand. If this is your first baby, the changes will be very noticeable to you.

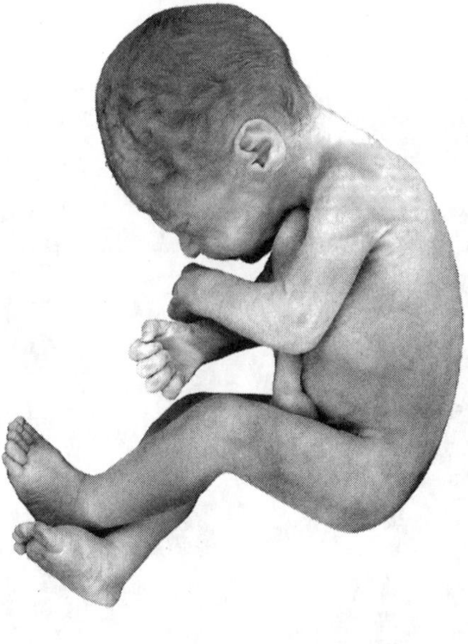

Notes:

....

....

The baby's eyes re-open now. It can see diffuse pinkish-red light through your abdomen. The cerebral cortex is composed of six cellular layers, just like an adult's. Specific layers of the cerebral cortex receive input from the various senses and some of these cells make contact in the spinal cord to directly cause muscle contractions, or movement. These neural circuits are responsible for purposeful movements, like visually-guided movements where the baby will reach for an object it sees. The cerebral cortex is responsible for many of the behaviors like speech and complex thought that apparently distinguish us as human.

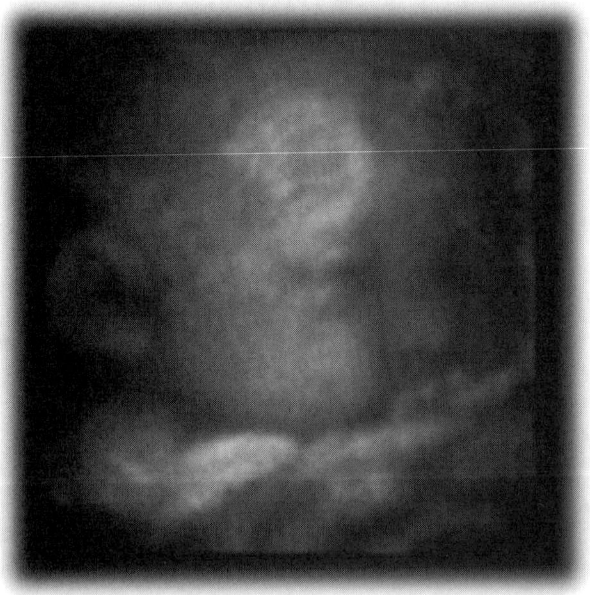

DAY 165

The baby is bathed in a rich chemosensory (taste and odor) environment. Odors are detected suspended in the amniotic fluid. In adults, all odor molecules must first be 'wet' by the nasal mucosa before we can 'smell' them. The aquatic olfactory environment, while different from an adult's experience, must be a very rich and interesting one. The circular fibers of the iris form, enabling the pupil to constrict and dilate. The visual part of the cerebral cortex - the occipital lobe - experiences dramatic growth these weeks.

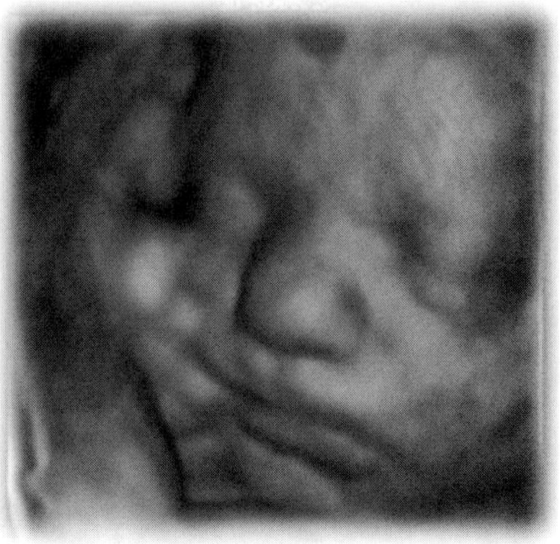

Notes:

....

....

DAY 166

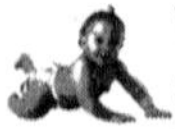

What is the baby 'smelling or tasting?' Fluid-borne substances reach the chemoreceptors by the constant regeneration of amniotic fluid and perfusion of the fluid through the nasal cavity. When you eat or drink something, various chemical cues reach your baby. In one experiment, pregnant women drank two cups of coffee. One group of women drank decaffeinated, the other drank regular caffeinated coffee. Real-time recordings of fetal activity found that both groups of fetuses showed increased heart rate responses and increased breathing rate after their mothers drank the coffee. Factors other than the caffeine present in the coffee caused the behavioral changes in the fetus. The babies are detecting something in the coffee and responding to it.

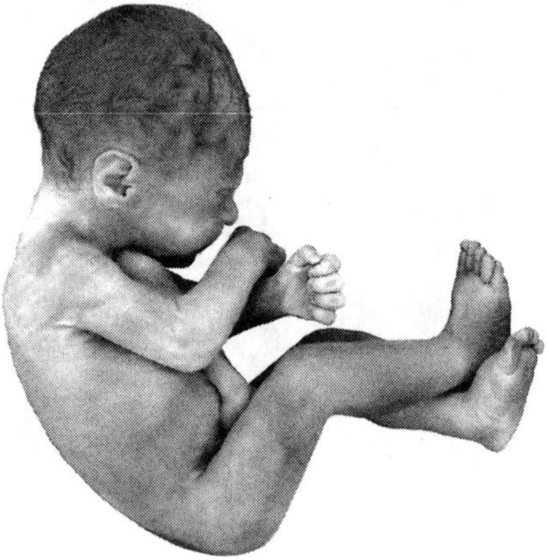

Thoughts:

....

....

DAY 167

Alterations of blood flow through the placenta and umbilical cord can alter the chemical composition of the amniotic fluid enough that the baby can remember it after birth. For example, maternal smoking produces a transitory decrease in placental blood flow. In animal experiments using rats, scientists can reduce blood flow to the fetus by briefly compressing the cord...at the same time they place an orange-flavored substance into the amniotic fluid. Another group of pups receives the cord clamping procedure but no orange substance. After these rat pups are born, the group exposed to the clamping and the orange taste will avoid the orange taste whereas rat pups exposed to the cord clamping alone will not avoid the orange taste. The implication is that the temporary decrease in blood flow (leading to decreased oxygen) is unpleasant and the orange taste that was present was linked to the unpleasant state. In humans, perhaps mothers who smoke are more likely to have babies that are finicky eaters.

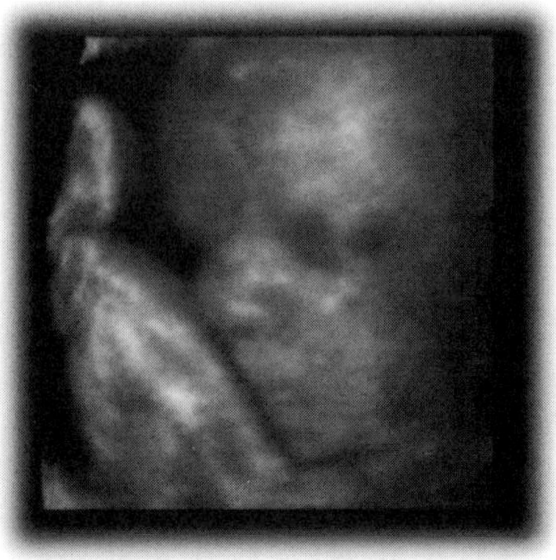

DAY 168

Your baby can also directly influence the chemical composition of the amniotic environment. Urea is an ammonia-like compound present in the urine the baby releases. Near full-term babies will release about 51 ml of urine per hour. Metabolites of wheat can be detected in amniotic fluid if the mother eats bread. Smells of cumin, fenugreek, garlic and curry can easily be detected in amniotic fluid collected from a woman who has recently consumed these spices. Some scientists believe that with a sufficiently sensitive detection method that you could demonstrate transfer to the fetus of all circulating tastes and 'smells'.

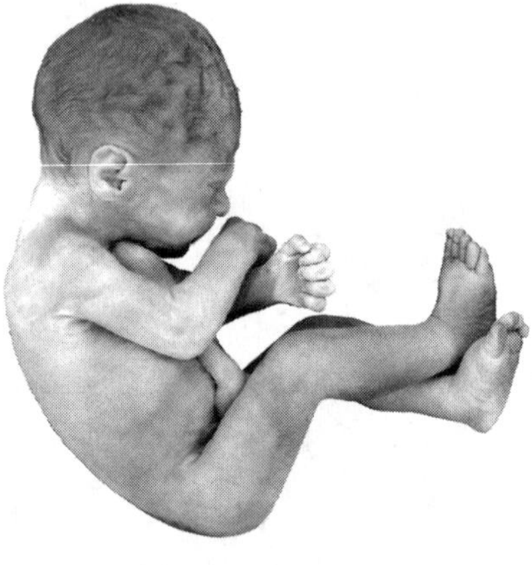

Thoughts:

....

....

DAY 169

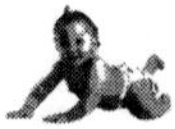

It's the beginning of the 7th month of your pregnancy. Your baby is about 14-1/4 inches long and weighs about 2 pounds. The longest bone in the body - the thigh bone or femur - continues to ossify. The femur hardens sooner in female babies, another sex-related difference.

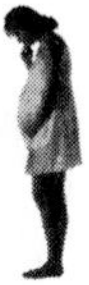

This month's checkup will involve weight and blood pressure, urine sample, fetal heartbeat, fetal size, measurement of the size and shape of your uterus and a general exam.

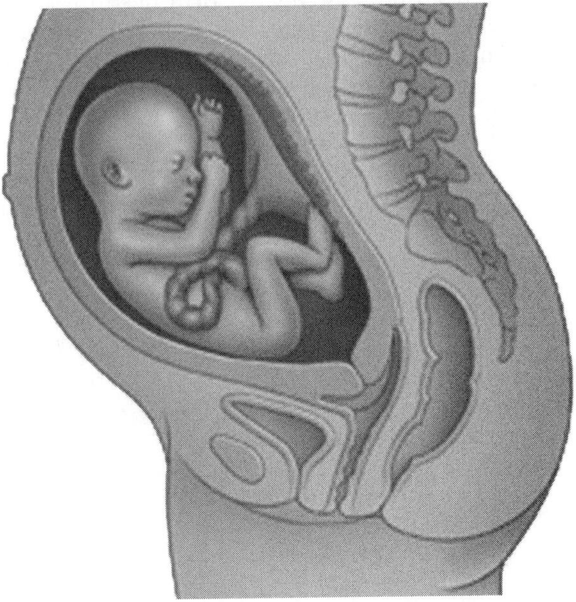

Notes:

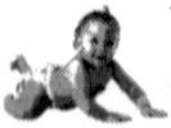

Your baby's brain is taking on a more mature look with the development of characteristic grooves and valleys called fissures and sulci. As the neurons grow they are assembled in regions that control and generate all of our behavior. Specific regions of the brain control specific behaviors. For example, the area labeled below is the main cortical area involved in auditory perception - hearing.

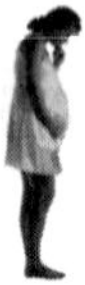

Because of all the changes in your blood volume and increased workload on your heart, you'll need to be careful when standing up. Rising too fast or bending down suddenly can make you light-headed and even possibly faint. Move slowly and deliberately so your cardiovascular system keeps pace.

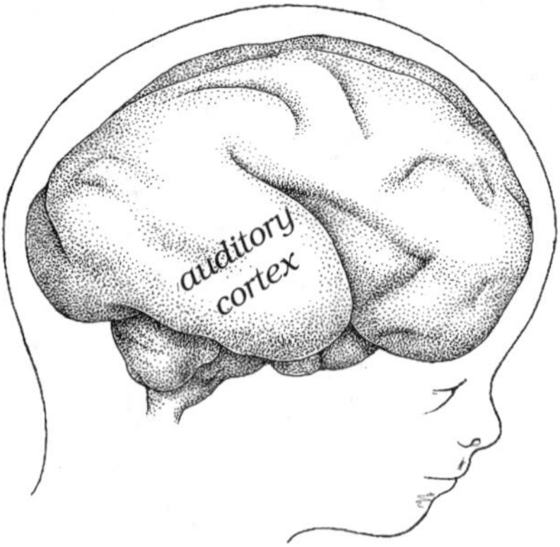

from Cowan (1977)

Thoughts:

....

....

DAY 171

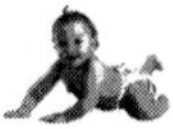

Your baby will fill out this month packing on fat. This will cause your baby to lose its wrinkled appearance as its skin is smoothed out by the underlying fat. By next month, about 4% of its entire weight will be white fat - the type of fat used for energy and body heat regulation.

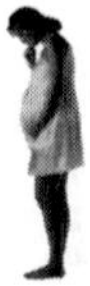

Choosing a birthing class: Many new parents opt to attend a class to help prepare them for labor and delivery. Check around with family and friends to see what classes they took and whether they found them useful.

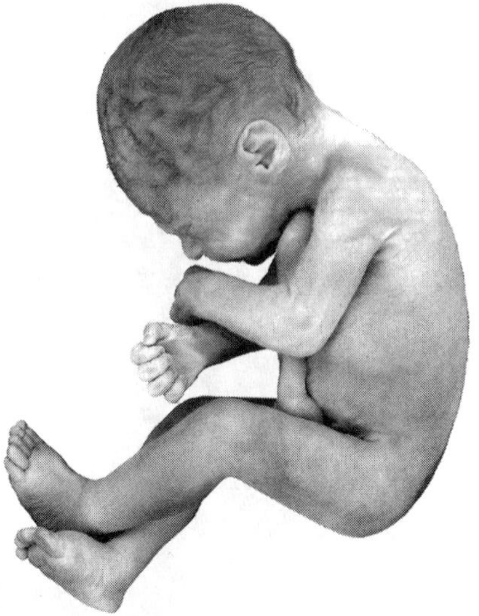

Notes:

....

....

DAY 172

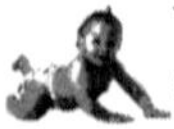

You're not wasting your time speaking to your baby. A variety of studies have shown that babies of this age will respond *in utero* to female and male voices with a deceleration or decrease in heart rate. They orient to the sound and the behavior of the heart indicates that they are listening. Kids actually listening and paying attention when you speak...enjoy it while it lasts!

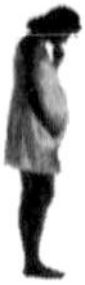

People tend to have a fear of the unknown. Birth is no different. The purpose of a birth preparation class is to inform you as to what to expect and this information should reduce the anxiety or fear that accompanies the unknown.

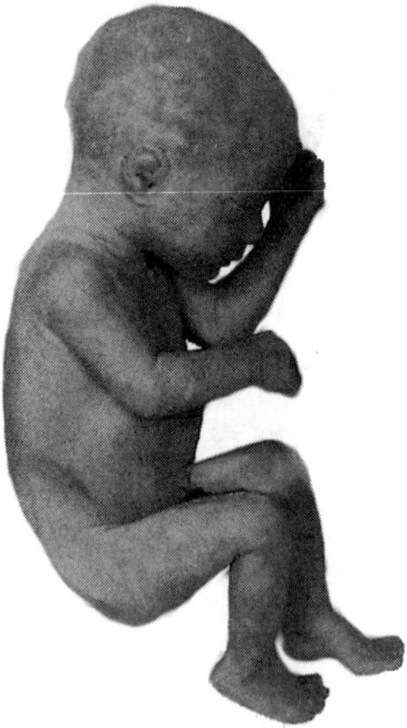

Thoughts:

....

....

DAY 173

The acoustic environment of the womb is filled with lots of sounds. Some sounds are more common in terms of frequency, like the mother's voice and heart beat, as well as intensity, like the mother's voice and heart beat. Newborn babies like prose spoken by a female voice, a solo female singing voice, a group of females singing and heart beat sounds. As for male speech and purely instrumental music, babies can take it or leave it. And white noise (a hissing sound) and the sounds of a heart beating faster than normal is upsetting to babies.

The critical difference between preferred and non-preferred sounds is whether the baby experienced them *in utero.* You might say that *familiarity breeds content.*

* *for a explanation of how scientists demonstrate that babies prefer certain sounds over others, refer to the glossary under* Non-nutritive sucking paradigm.

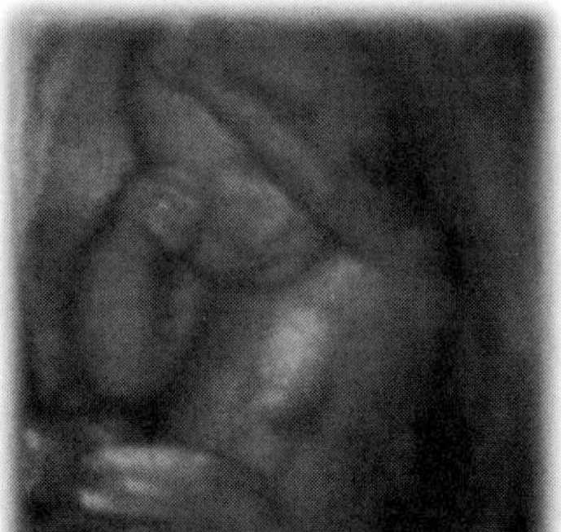

Stretching 3D ultrasound image

Notes:

....

....

DAY 174

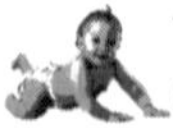

Your baby is not simply a passive listener. They have very clear *preferences* for certain sounds over others. Newborn babies prefer:*

- their own mother's voice vs. other females
- female voices vs. male voices
- the sound of a heart beat vs. male voices
- no preference for father's voice vs. other males (*sorry dad!*)

How can a newborn prefer some sounds over others? Prenatal experience, learning and memory.

*refer to page 274 for further explanation of how preferences are demonstrated in babies.

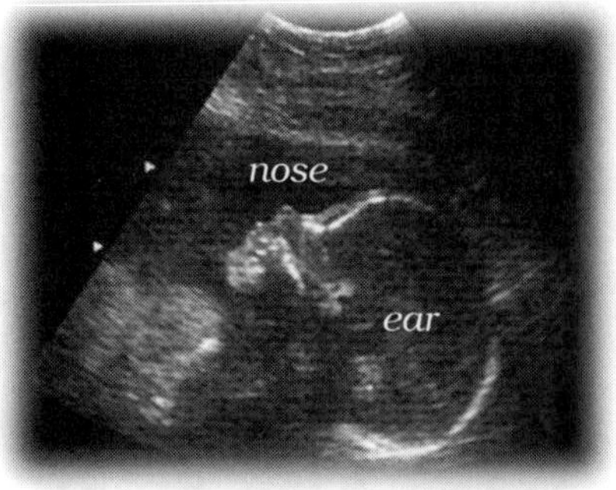

Profile

Thoughts:

....

....

DAY 175

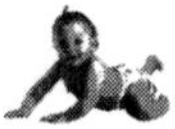

Your baby will inhale twice as much amniotic fluid as it will swallow. It is practicing breathing - exercising the breathing muscles and diaphragm, helping them to work together in a coordinated manner. Interestingly, this practice occurs only during REM sleep. In adults, studies have found that some brainstem respiratory centers that monitor oxygen saturation in the blood may temporarily reduce functioning during REM sleep. This increased respiration, which is a defining feature of REM sleep in adults, may be the body's way of ensuring adequate oxygen levels during this period of neural blackout. Better to breathe too much than not enough.

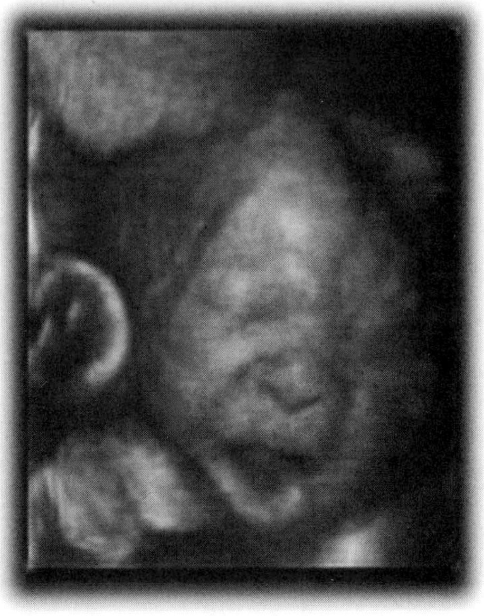

Structures that detect pressure, known as Pacinian corpuscles, embedded deep in the skin are fully formed and functional in the fingers. Your baby also has all the free nerve endings (pain receptors) hooked up and working in the finger tips now. As the fingers increase in size during childhood and adolescence, the number of free nerve endings doesn't increase. Instead, they are stretched thinner and spread out over a wider surface area. Can this anatomical difference be involved in the widely different response of a child vs. an adult to a minor injury? Perhaps the spreading out of pain receptive sensors with growth produces fewer pain signals to the brain, so the same injury really doesn't hurt as bad to an adult.
Baby is 15-1/4 inches ❦ 2.4 lbs.

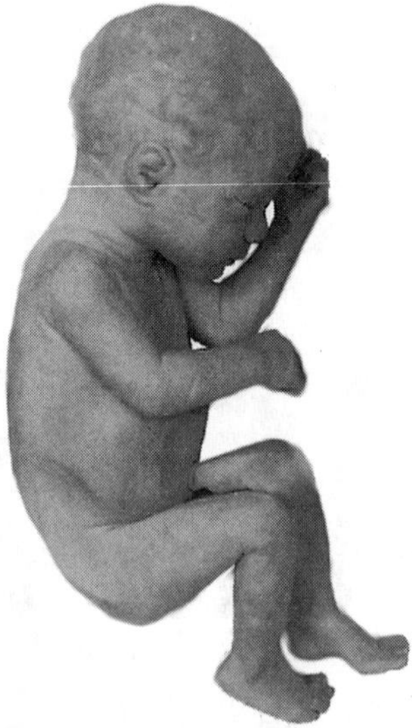

Thoughts:

....

....

DAY 177

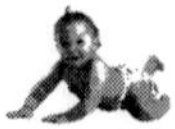

Your baby's skin has taken on its color by the addition and final migration of cells called melanocytes. These cells produce melanin that contribute pigment or color to the skin. Sweat glands are now present in the skin as well.

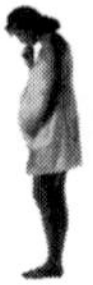

Aspirin should be avoided, unless directed by your doctor. Aspirin works by blocking prostaglandins which are involved in the transmission of pain signals. Prostaglandins are involved in the labor process as well so aspirin can have an adverse effect upon the normal labor and delivery process.

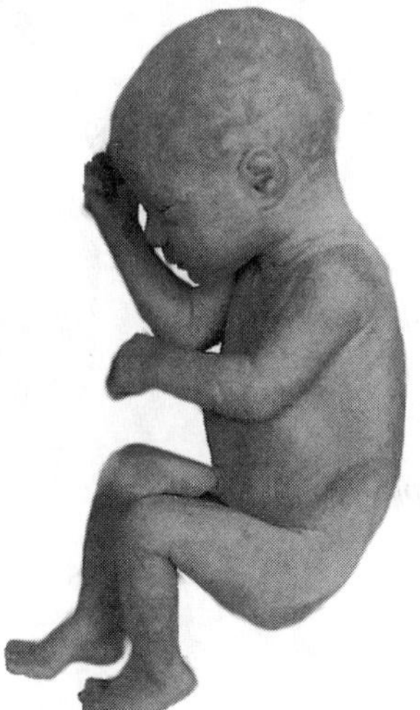

Notes:

....

....

DAY 178

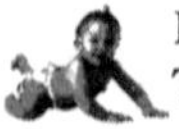

By now all of the areas of the skin are responsive to touch. The last area of the body to become sensitive to touch (measured by the baby's movement in response to) is the inside of the nostrils. Sneezing is possible now because the sensory component of the reflex is in place.

Area	*When responsive to touch (week)*
Upper lip	*5.5 weeks*
Nose & chin	*7*
Bridge of nose, eyelid	*8.5*
Palms	*8.5*
Genital areas	*8.5*
Shoulder	*8.5*
Soles of feet	*9*
Eyebrows & forehead	*9*
Upper arm & forearm	*9*
Back	*9*
Upper chest	*9.5*
Thighs & legs	*10*
Rest of chest	*11*
Front part of tongue	*12*
Shoulder blades	*12*
Abdomen	*13*
Buttocks	*15*
External ear - pinna	*15.5*
Back of hand	*16.5*
Back of tongue	*16.5 weeks*

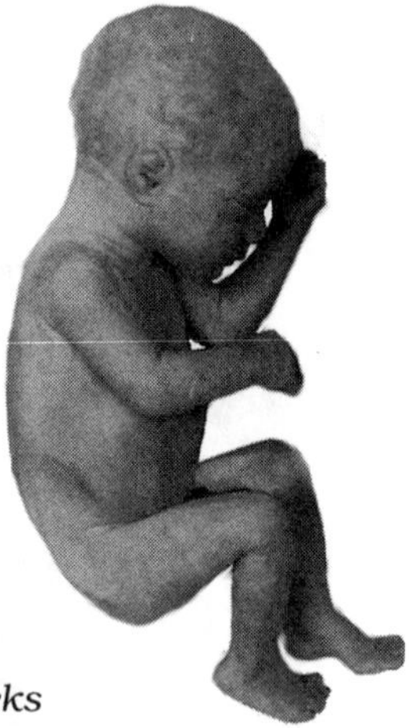

Thoughts:

....

....

DAY 179

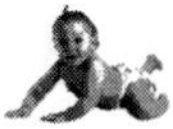

Read your baby a story now and it could be its favorite later. In an experiment, mothers read passages of the *Cat in the Hat* or *The King, The Mice and The Cheese* twice each day when they could feel that their 7.5 month old fetus was awake. They did this every day until birth. Another group of babies were not read the stories. Two days after birth, the babies were played recordings of their mother or another female reading the familiar passage, or their mother reading the unfamiliar passage. Babies suck more during events they like or prefer. Babies who had been read the passages from 7.5 months on sucked more than babies not read to, and they also sucked more during the familiar passage compared to the unfamiliar one...even if the familiar passage was read to them by another female. *More>>>*

3D Ultrasound
showing face and feet

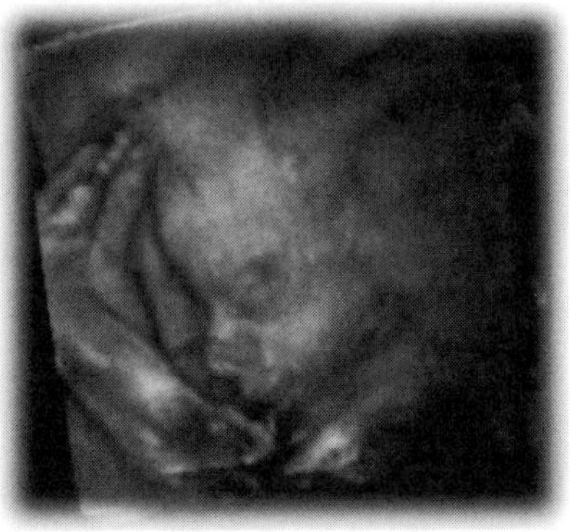

Notes:

....

....

DAY 180

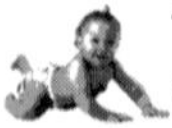

This study demonstrates that it is the content of the passage - not their mother - that the baby is responding to. The group of babies that was first read the passage after birth didn't show a preference for either passage. This study also shows that babies prefer what is familiar to them and that they learn and remember complex sounds they experienced prenatally.

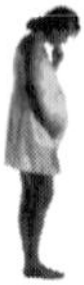

There are three main types or philosophies of prenatal classes. They are the Grantly Dick-Read Method; the Lamaze Method and the Bradley Method.

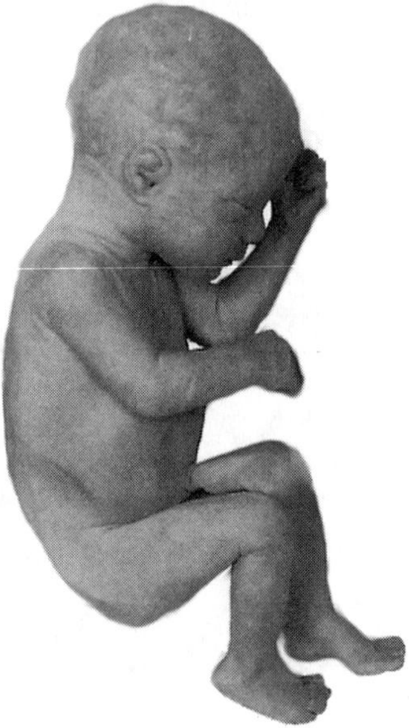

Thoughts:

....

....

DAY 181

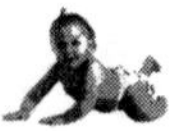

Many babies will take an upside-down position in the uterus, positioning their head in your pelvis. Over the next 6 weeks or so the baby's head will press on the cervix and before birth the cervix will flatten or efface. Cervix means 'neck' in latin.

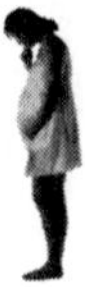

The Grantly Dick-Read approach combines relaxation techniques and prenatal education to de-mystify the labor process. When you know what to expect, uncertainty decreases and so should anxiety. This method was the first to incorporate fathers into the birth process and allow them into the delivery room.

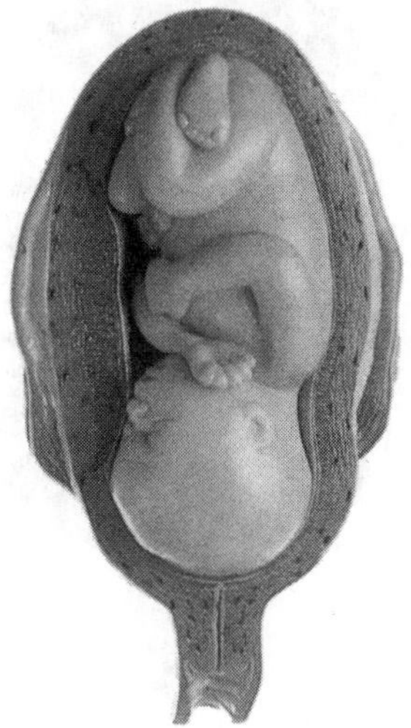

Notes:

....

....

If you're carrying twins they could be positioned like this. One head-up; the other head-down. Twin heart beats can be detected because they will be slightly out of phase with each other, too fast to be a single heart beating.

The Lamaze method combines knowledge with relaxation training to help de-mystify birth and alleviate pain. Lamaze involves conditioning or training the mother to perform useful responses like controlled regulated breathing to help alleviate labor pains. The father or coach trains with the mother to assist her during the birth.

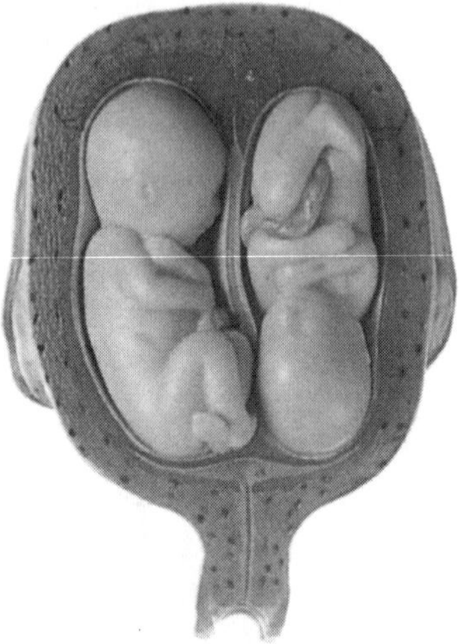

Thoughts:

....

....

DAY 183

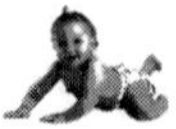

Your baby is acquiring cues from its native language now. Since the transfer of your voice is so clear, it can learn and incorporate characteristics of your voice. Using acoustic spectroscopy - which generates a 'sound fingerprint' of a voice - the cry of a 27-week old prematurely born baby contains some of the speech features, rhythms and characteristics of the mother. This is yet another example of prenatal learning.

Baby is 15 inches ❦ 2-1/2 lbs.

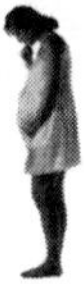

The Bradley method emphasizes exercise and diet as the best means to prepare for the rigors of birth. Accordingly, Bradley classes start earlier than the last trimester. This method originated the father-coached delivery. Rather than panting exercises to control the pain of contractions, the Bradley method emphasizes deep abdominal breathing to divert attention from the contractions to the processes involved in taking a deep breath.

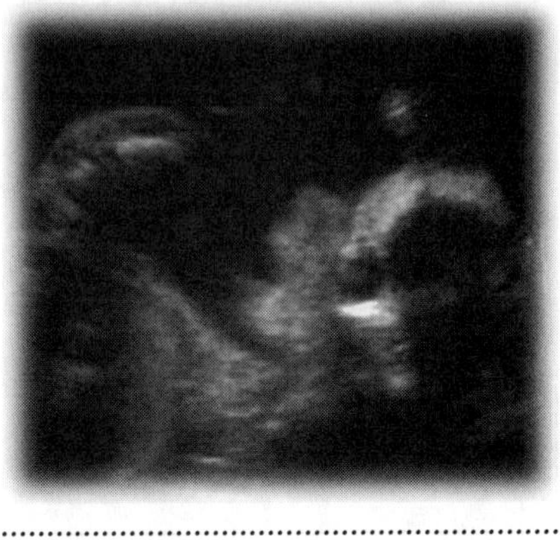

Notes:

....

....

DAY 184

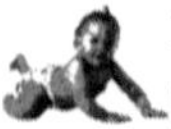

Much of the research on prenatal learning examines the responses of newborns. If the newborn shows a specific behavior it is considered as evidence of prenatal learning (since presumable the baby hasn't has the opportunity to learn the response in the short time she has been out of the womb). Having said that...newborns prefer speech sounds of their mother's native language heard *in utero*. English newborns prefer to look at people speaking English; French babies prefer French, and so on.

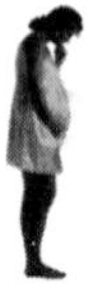

Each of your breasts will gain about 1-1/2 pounds by birth in preparation for breast feeding.

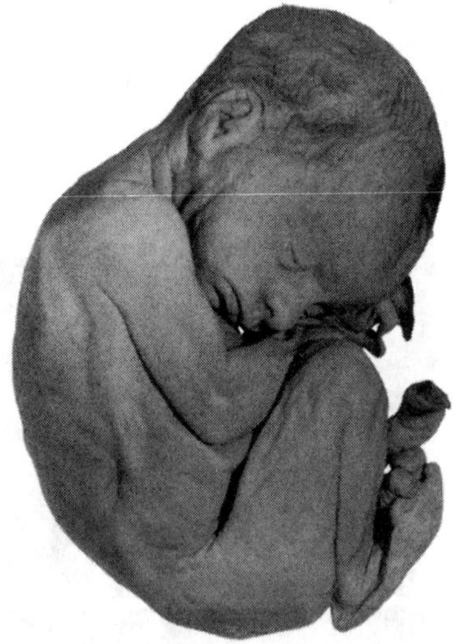

Thoughts:

....

....

DAY 185

<u>Where the weight comes from during pregnancy</u>

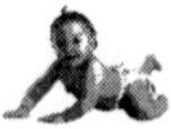

About 26 pounds is the average amount of overall weight gain during a normal pregnancy. Below is the breakdown of where that weight comes from.

Weight of baby	7.50 lbs
Weight of placenta	1.50 lbs
Weight of amniotic fluid	1.75 lbs
Increase in weight of breasts & uterus	3.0 lbs
Blood volume & fluid	5.25lbs
Maternal fat	7.0 lbs
	26 lbs

Most women will gain an average of 11 pounds in the last trimester. On average, about 2400 calories per day is required during the last trimester.

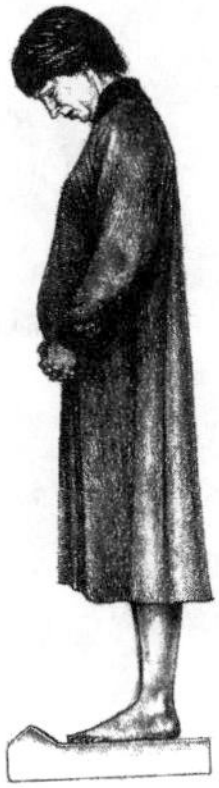

Notes:

....

....

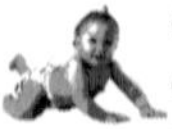

Can a baby feel and express emotion at this age? 27-week old premature babies show the same facial reactions as adults to odors and tastes. Give a pleasant taste like strawberry, banana or vanilla and the baby will turn her head toward the taste and make a facial reaction that looks like she is pleased. She will turn her head away from fishy or rotten tastes and make a face that is associated with disgust. Yucky!

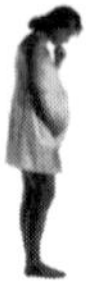

Some women normally experience leaking fluid from their breasts during the last trimester. This fluid known as colostrum, or pre-milk, contains antibodies and protein. This will help protect and nourish your baby in the first few days after birth.

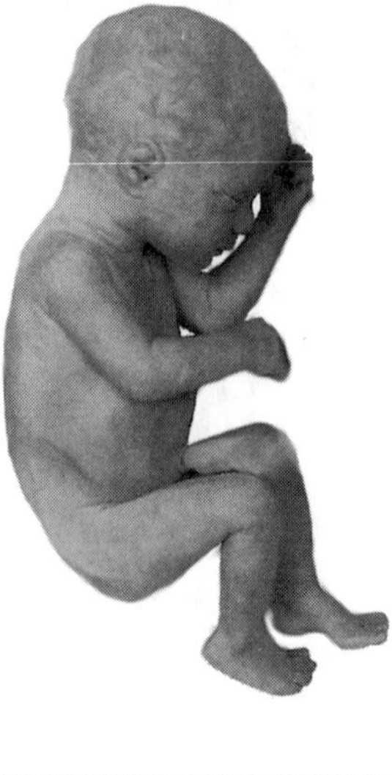

Thoughts:

....

....

DAY 187

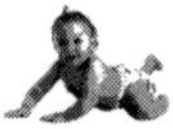

Ultrasound analyses and observation of premature babies shows that they smile now...particularly during REM sleep. The adaptive value of a facial movement like smiling on caregivers can't be underestimated.

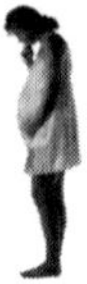

The vast majority of the iron that will be stored in your baby's liver will be transferred from you to your baby now. Make sure that you maintain your iron intake. The stored iron will be drawn upon by your baby during the first few months of life, since milk provides little iron to the baby.

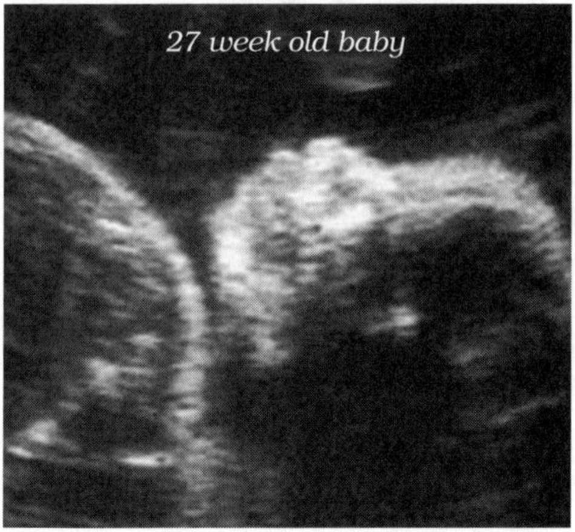

27 week old baby

Notes:

....

....

DAY 188

The general activity level and movement of your baby will start to decrease now. Early in development (around 12 weeks) periods of inactivity are relatively rare - the baby is moving constantly - rarely is there a period of more than 10 minutes without movement. Now there are periods of inactivity - lasting up to 45 minutes. This reflects maturation of parts of the brain that reduce, or inhibit, neural activity. In the case of movement, your baby can actively stop moving. This is a hallmark of more mature neural functioning.

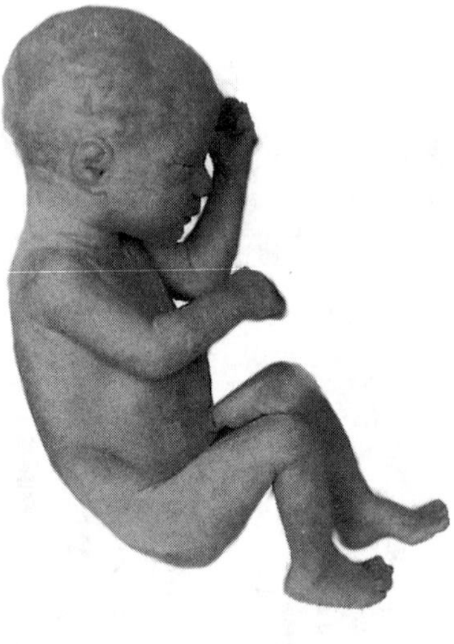

Thoughts:

....

....

DAY 189

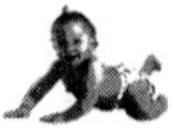

Slowing of the heart rate in response to a sound is a measure of attention and cognitive processing. The heart rate orienting response occurs during both quiet (non-REM) and REM sleep now. The orienting response is more pronounced in quiet sleep, and girls show a significantly greater orienting response to a sound at this age than do boy babies.

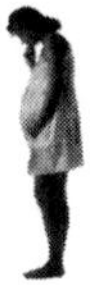

Some women experience unusual dreams during their pregnancy. Dreams typically incorporate the happenings of the day into their content. Having a baby is a big, life-changing event, it's only fitting that your dreams reflect your thoughts and feelings about your baby and being a mother.

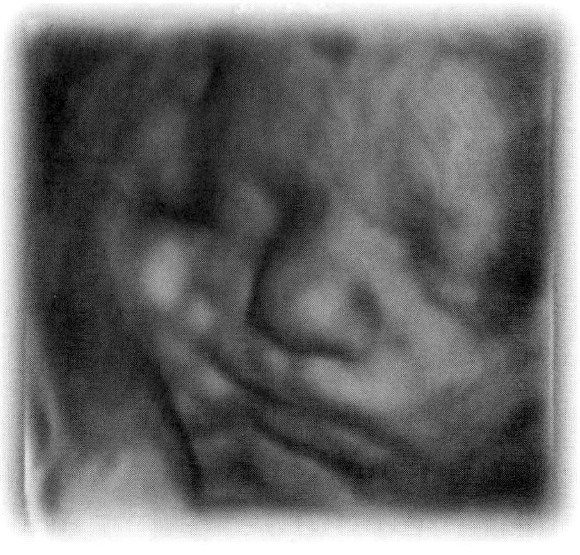

DAY 190

By now your baby will be opening and shutting its eyes regularly. But what is it looking at? Even the brightest of lights are diffusely transmitted through the abdominal wall. The best example of what your baby sees is to shine a flashlight through your hand...only a diffuse red light and glow. Babies can see and will track or follow a light placed on the abdomen. Real-time ultrasound examinations enable scientists to try these simple experiments on babies and observe their responses.

Baby is 17 inches ❦ 3.0 lbs.

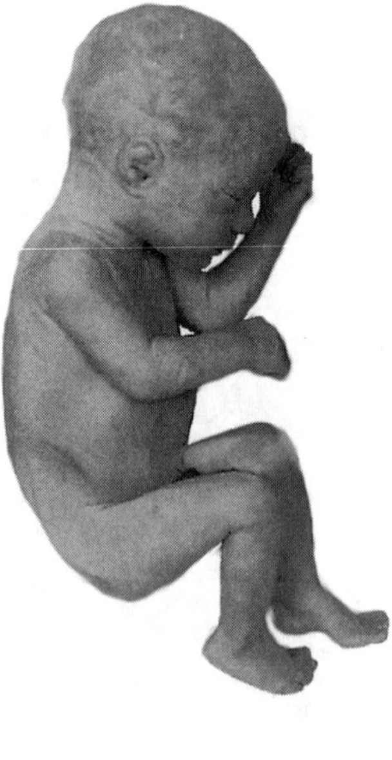

Thoughts:

....

....

DAY 191

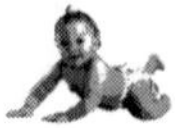

In the nearly lightless environment of the womb how can the eyes function at birth with virtually no prior experience? The answer is another clever twist of nature. The retina - the light sensitive area in the back of the eye - creates its own signals now that 'program' the visual part of the brain to respond to light signals in the appropriate way. This way when the baby is born into the outside, visually dominant, light-filled environment, the visual system is ready to function.

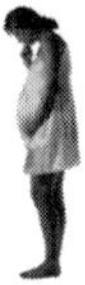

A new baby is born once every 8 seconds in the United States - that's over 10,000 per day! Your 8 seconds is only a couple of months away.

Profile showing thumb sucking

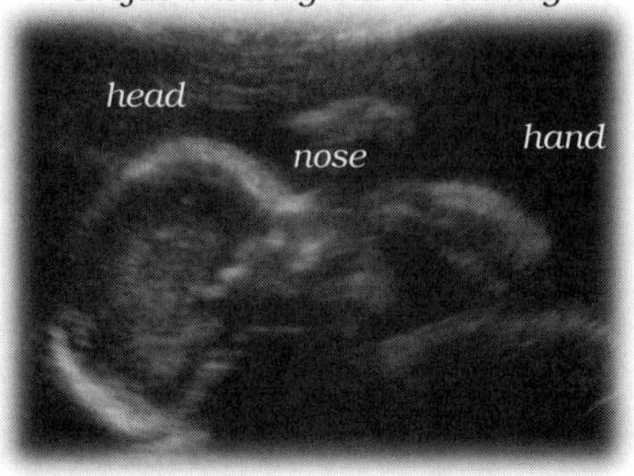

Notes:

....

....

DAY 192

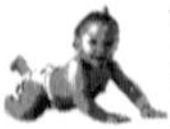

Your baby's teeth are hooked up to their nerves, with the tooth pulp and enamel enveloping the nerve. Located just to the side of the baby tooth is a bud for a permanent tooth. Babies have 20 teeth; adults have 32. By 6 months after birth, this permanent tooth bud will migrate and embed itself under the erupting milk tooth, then wait 5 - 15 years until it is due to emerge from the gum.

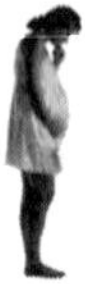

You can travel by air up to the 36th Week. As you get larger you'll find it more cumbersome to navigate around the cramp seats and you'll want to get up and stroll the isles. After the 36th Week, commercial airlines may ask you when you're due...they don't want you going into labor mid-flight.

3D ultrasound of face

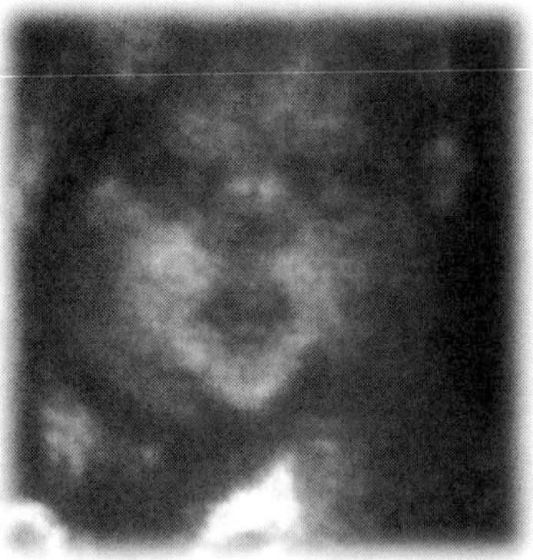

Thoughts:

....

....

DAY 193

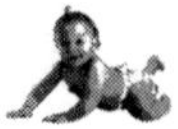

Babies show distinct behavioral states. Just as adults cycle between wake and sleep, your baby has four defined states that are consistent from baby to baby.

> <u>State 1F</u> - quiet, still state which can be interrupted by brief whole body movements and startles. No eye movements; heart rate is stable. There are also mouthing movements.
> <u>State 2F</u> - frequent movements; stretching and arm and leg movement. Eye movement and heart rate increases during movements.
> <u>State 3F</u> - No whole body movements. Eye movement present; no heart rate changes. Sucking movements commonly seen.
> <u>State 4F</u> - Vigorous continuous activity. Eye movements; heart rate increases.

Consideration of the baby's behavioral state is important for the proper interpretation of psychological experiments. For example, babies are more responsive to sounds when they are quiet and awake (State 1F). Lack of a response without determination of the baby's state may just mean that the baby was sleeping.

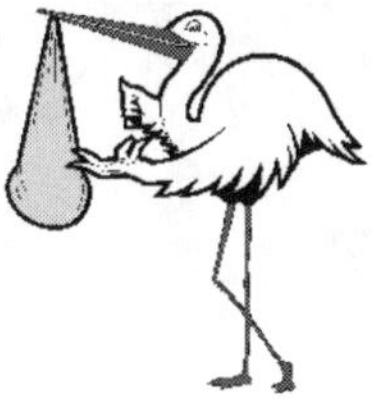

Notes:

....

....

DAY 194

Babies are commonly seen with their hands held close to their mouths. Less common is a view showing the baby actually sucking its thumb. The general activity shown by your baby is more than just exercise. Studies with animals have demonstrated that restriction of fetal movement for as short as a day will permanently impair the range of movement shown later.

One new financial consideration that many first-time parents have is life insurance. Since it can take a month or longer from the time you contact the insurer until the policy goes into effect, planning ahead is wise. A blood and urine sample will need to be taken (usually at your home), and a nurse will measure your vital signs.

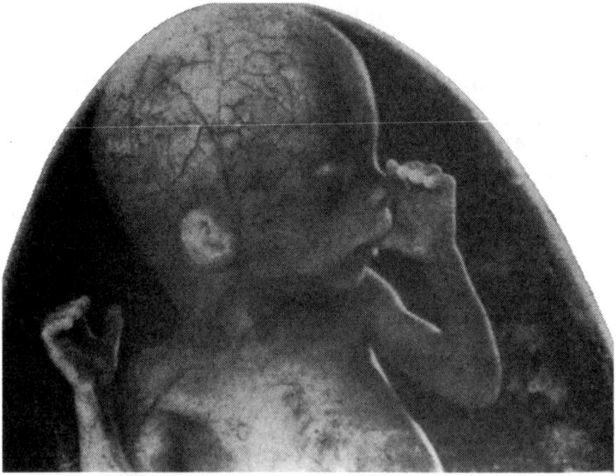

Thoughts:

....

....

DAY 195

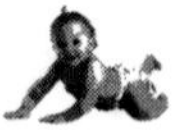

The baby's skin is semi-transparent, with many of the larger blood vessels clearly visible through the skin. Over the next few weeks the final layers of the skin will develop, adding thickness, more hair and more pigment.

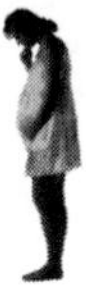

The likelihood of having twins is about 1 in 40. About two-third's of twins are identical twins (one fertilized egg that splits in two). The other third are fraternal twins (two eggs fertilized by separate sperm). If you're over 30, you have a greater chance of having twins because you're producing more hormones that stimulate ovulation, which could lead to multiple egg release. Also, taller women are about 30% more likely to have twins.

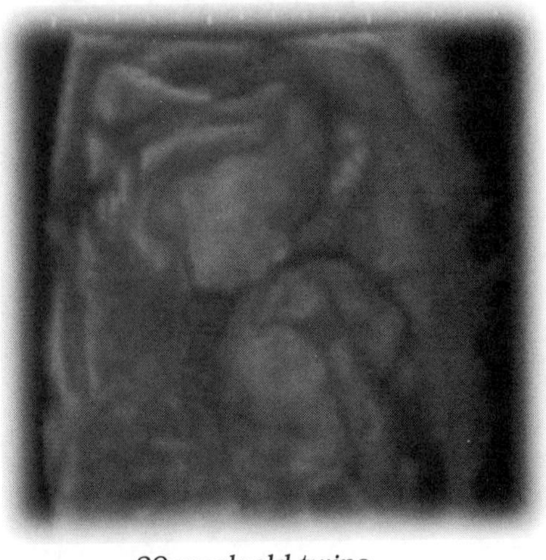

29 week old twins

Notes:

....

....

Just like babies show a preference for specific sounds, newborn and premature babies prefer to look at specific things as well. For example, in a preferential looking test, newborns look longer at patterns than they do at non-patterned images. The pattern they like to look at the longest is the human face. Since they haven't had much experience looking at faces in the womb, these findings suggest a pre-wired, innate process that directs the baby's gaze and attention to a face. Some researchers think this behavior elicits protective behavior from the parents and may help foster infant-caregiver bonding.

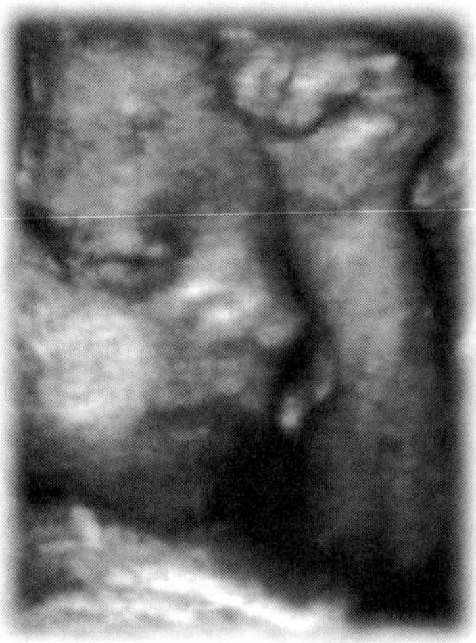

Thoughts:

....

....

DAY 197

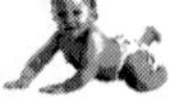

This is the beginning of the last two months...you're rounding third base, heading for home! Your baby is really growing. It is 18 inches ❦ 3-1/2 lbs.

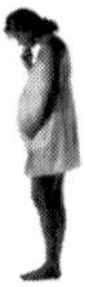

This month's checkup will involve weight and blood pressure measurement, urine sample, fetal heartbeat, fetal size, measurement of the size and shape of your uterus and a general exam.

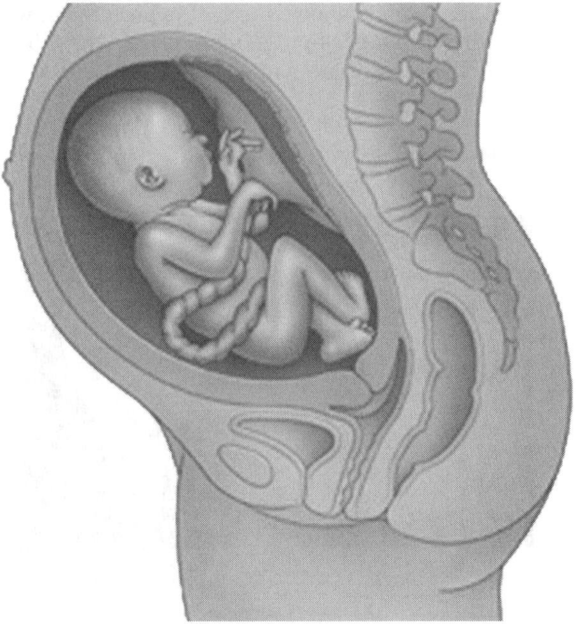

Notes:

....

....

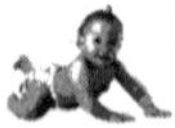

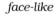

Babies prefer to look at faces. Amazing studies have teased apart the reasons why babies show this preference. It is the configuration of the facial elements (the specific position of the eyes and mouth) that babies are attending to. Babies prefer to look at the face-like configuration on the left (which has the eyes and mouth properly positioned) but not the figure on the right. This study indicates that babies possess a brain mechanism specifically tuned or wired to respond to structural information conveyed by a face-like pattern. Further studies showed that this preference was governed by very early developing , more primitive, *sub*-cortical visual structures, not later maturing visual cortical structures.

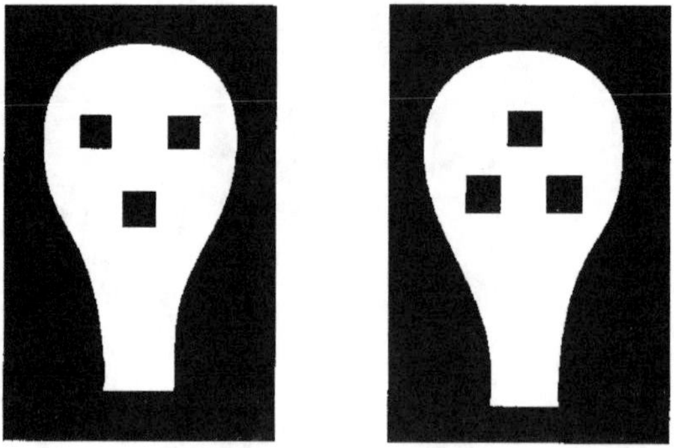

face-like *non face-like*

babies prefer to look at the face-like configuration compared to the figure (with equivalent but jumbled elements)

from Simion, Valenza & Umilta (1998)

DAY 199

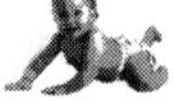

Body temperature can be controlled and regulated now. Rather than relying on the constant temperature of the amniotic bath to keep the baby's body temperature in a narrow range, internal control of the processes that influence temperature occur through the hypothalamus (a complex region in the base of the brain). Cooling and warming the body involves a coordination of sensory and vasomotor responses. As core body temperature rises, signals from the hypothalamus cause capillaries to dilate to disperse heat and cool the blood, and sweating occurs to cool the skin. If it's cold, shivering causes heat retention by raising body hair to trap heat, and capillary blood flow is redirected to the body core.

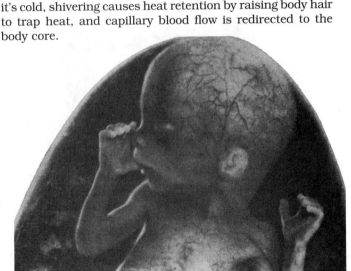

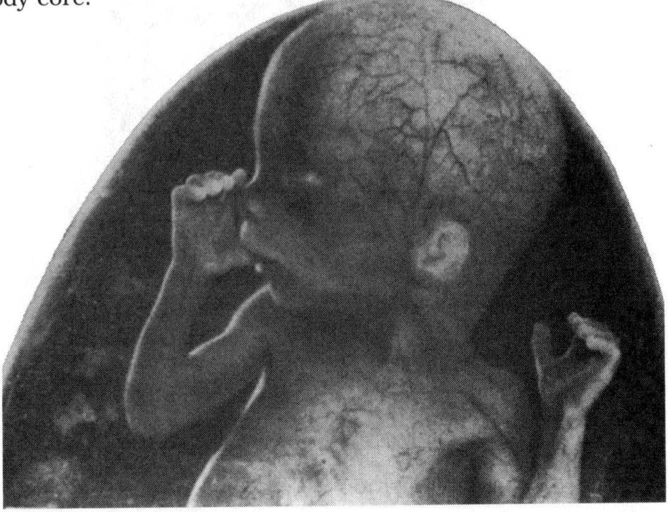

Notes:

....

....

One reliable predictor of later intelligence is the rate at which a baby habituates. When babies see something new, they look at it. Show the same thing again and again, over and over, and the baby will look less and less. The rate at which they get bored (look less) is a measure of attentional processing and habituation. Babies that are faster at extracting the information from a new image, then move on to soak up information from a new source tend to score higher on IQ tests at 2 years and 7.5 years of age. Habituation rate aside, still the best predictor of a child's IQ is genetics - the mother's and father's IQ.

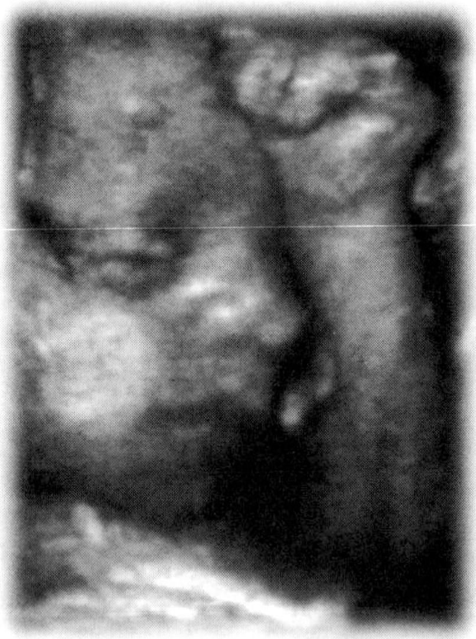

Thoughts:

....

....

DAY 201

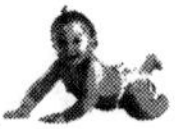

Boys and girls show some behavioral differences at this age. For example, girls will respond earlier to sound, with a deceleration in heart rate, compared to boys. The brains of boys and girls are also visibly different prenatally as well. Some of the structures - particularly in the hypothalamus, which organizes and controls sexual behavior - are visibly different to the naked eye. When examined under a microscope, the fine structure of the neurons and connections are radically different. These anatomical differences may underlie many behavioral differences.

A wave from a 29-wk old baby

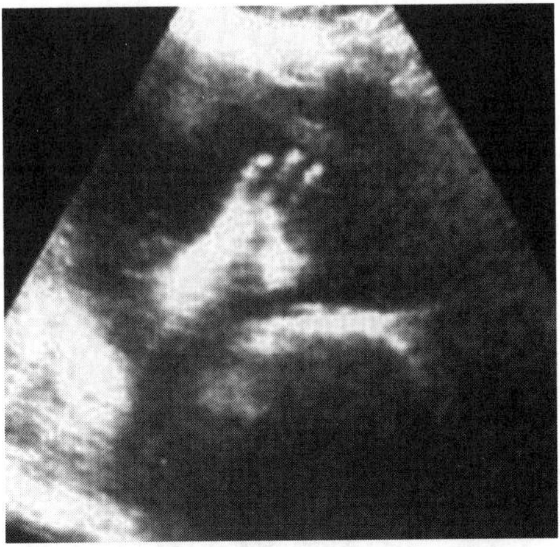

Notes:

....

....

DAY 202

Respiratory movements such as breathing, sighs, gasping and hiccups peak now and will diminish in frequency as birth approaches. During the last weeks of pregnancy, breathing movements can be absent for up to 2 hours...this is normal, and indicates the maturation of the nervous system. Eye movements can be observed during some ultrasound examinations.

Aspirin is also to be avoided when nursing. As much as 4% of the aspirin you ingest transfers to your milk. Aspirin is harmful to babies as it has been shown to build up in their tissues. Aspirin is also associated with the development of Reye's syndrome, a serious condition affecting the liver and brain.

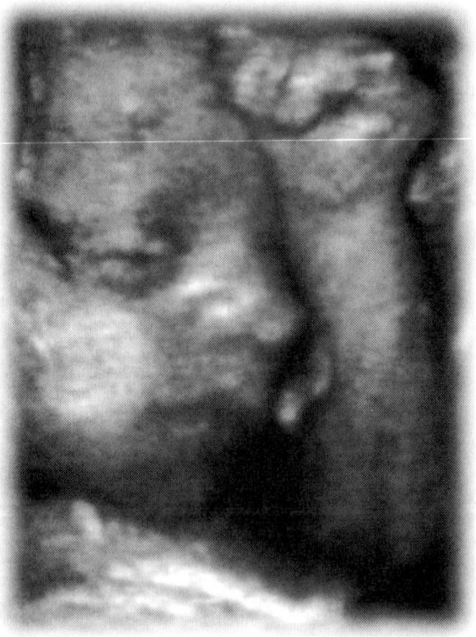

DAY 203

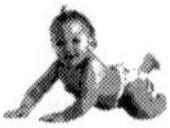

Your baby's resting heart rate will change during the course of development, showing a predictable, gradual decrease that will extend into childhood. At 16 weeks your baby's heart rate was about 155 beats/minute - it will decrease about 1 beat/minute each week until at birth when the resting heart rate is about 130 beats/minute. This decrease reflects the maturation of the cardiovascular system and resulting efficiencies in pumping blood throughout the body.

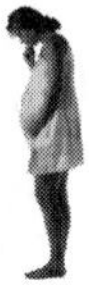

The incidence of episiotomy - a surgical procedure in which a small incision is made in the perineum to assist delivery and prevent tearing - has decreased in the United States. One study found that almost 70% of all vaginal births involved episiotomy in 1983. That rate dropped to just under 20% in 2000.

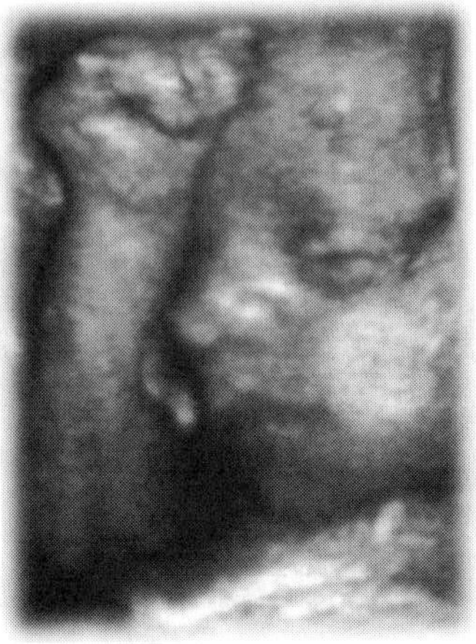

Notes:

....

....

DAY 204

Your baby spends a lot of its time hiccuping. At 14 weeks it was hiccuping more than 10% of the time, now it hiccups less than 2% of the time. This decrease in the frequency of hiccuping reflects maturation of the nervous system. What is the function of hiccups? No one knows for sure. Hiccups may be a neural artifact or leftover that may serve an important, though unknown, developmental need.

Baby is 19 inches ❦ 4.0 lbs.

There are a variety of birthmarks that can appear on your baby. Many babies have a reddish blotch at the base of the back of the neck or on the forehead. Some call these marks 'stork bites.' Also strawberries (hemangiomas), which appear as elevated red marks, can appear anywhere. Most of these marks fade and disappear by age 4 - 6.

Profile

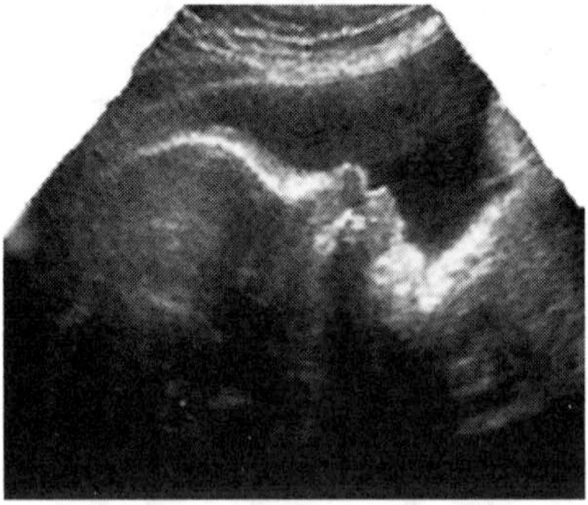

Thoughts:

....

....

DAY 205

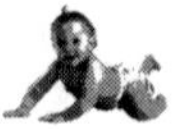

The amount of amniotic fluid surrounding your baby changes through the pregnancy.

10 weeks	30 ml
20 weeks	375 ml
30 weeks	850 ml

Your baby is ingesting about 750 ml of amniotic fluid per day. Nature must have a purpose for all this fluid ingestion and there are two recent discoveries that may provide clues. Amniotic fluid contains an - as yet unidentified - growth factor for the digestive tract. Animals studies have demonstrated that interference with amniotic fluid ingestion leads to underdeveloped stomachs and intestines. Also, amniotic fluid has nutritional value, primarily in the form of proteins and sugars. It is estimated that a third trimester baby gets 10-14% of its total daily nutrients from amniotic fluid.

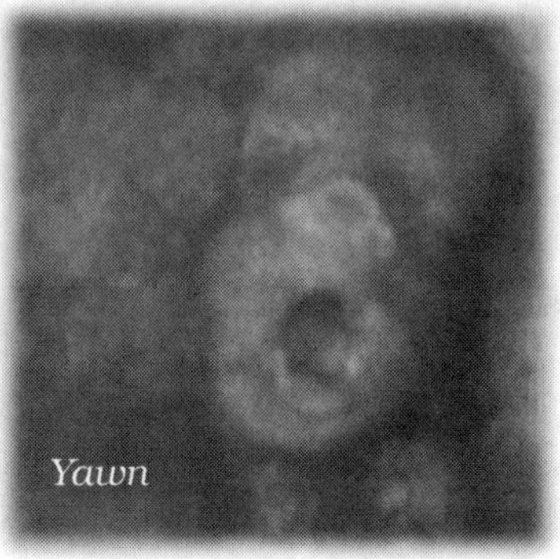

Yawn

Notes:

....

....

DAY 206

Smoking and drinking alcohol affects you and your baby. Alcohol ingestion results in a depression of breathing/swallowing movements in your baby that can last up to 30 minutes. Since the baby derives some nutrients from swallowing amniotic fluid they risk undernourishment. Animals experiments have demonstrated that high doses of alcohol decrease the amount of oxygen carried through the umbilical cord to the baby, essentially depriving the baby of oxygen. Alcohol has a variety of known effects on the fetus - none of them good. Smoking has similar effects. Alcohol suppresses the release of growth hormone from your baby's pituitary gland. Alcohol decreases cerebral protein synthesis, resulting in smaller brains, and malformed neurons. Fetal blood alcohol level is 20% higher than maternal blood levels because the baby lacks enzymes to metabolize alcohol.

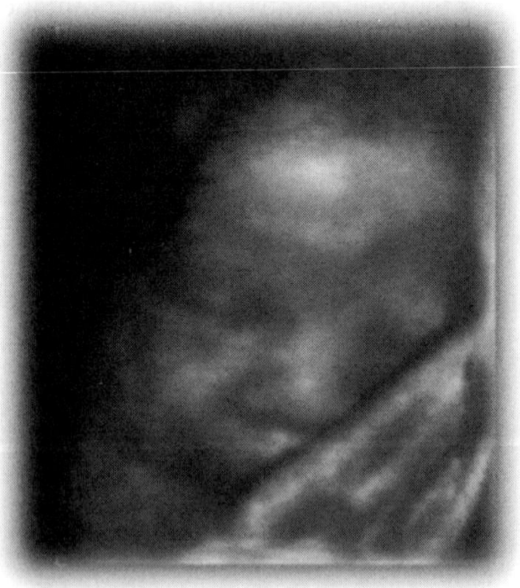

DAY 207

Babies show a variety of reflexes now, one of which is called the Moro reflex. In response to a loud noise or sudden loss of support (as if falling) a baby will reach forward with both arms as if grabbing for the mother for support. This reflex disappears 3 - 6 months after birth and appears to be actively inhibited or blocked by later maturing neural structures.

Braxton Hicks contractions are mild tensing or contractions of the uterine muscles. They occur for a short duration (30 - 60 seconds) and they are usually painless. Unlike true labor contractions, Braxton Hicks contractions don't increase in intensity, they are unpredictable and they don't occur with any periodicity (they are not rhythmic).

Moro reflex in newborn

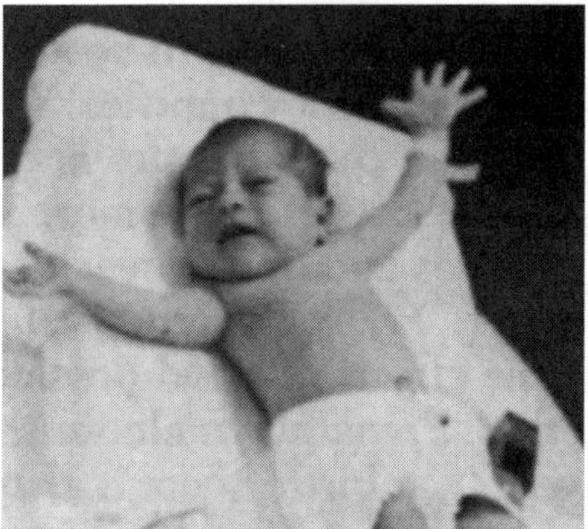

Notes:

....

....

DAY 208

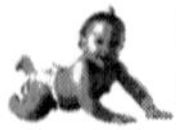

Reflexes that help your baby locate and acquire food are also present now. Sucking reflexes elicited by touching the lips are required for suckling. Rooting reflexes elicited by touching your baby's cheek cause the head to turn toward the source of stimulation...helpful in locating a nipple. When the time comes to nurse - don't push your baby's head toward the nipple. Your hand will cause your baby to reflexively root toward your hand and away from the nipple, making attachment difficult and subsequently frustrating both you and your baby.

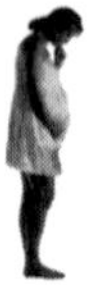

One function of Braxton Hicks -type contractions is to facilitate and increase blood circulation through the placenta during the last few weeks of pregnancy.

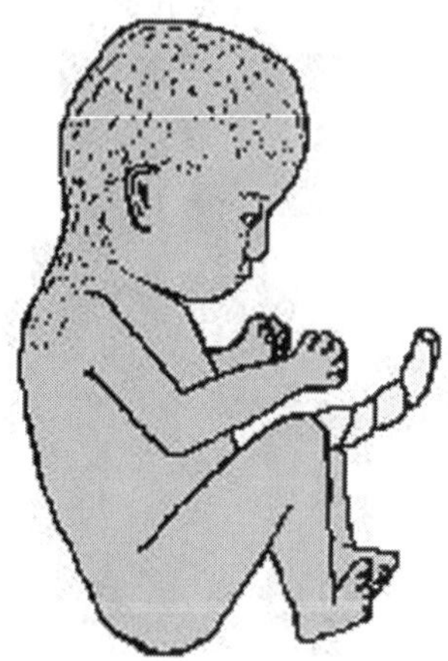

Thoughts:

....

....

Touching the sole of your baby's foot will cause the fanning or spreading out of the toes. This is the Babinski reflex. This reflex is gone about 4 - 6 months after birth and is replaced by the mature reflex which is a clenching of the toes downward in response to stroking the sole. Sometimes after a brain injury - like a stroke - the Babinski reflex will reappear. This demonstrates that the damaged neural structure was actively inhibiting the reflex.

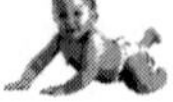

False labor contractions: Your uterus hardens and softens intermittently and typically only involves a portion of the uterus. False labor lacks a pattern: there is no rhythmicity or predictability. The contractions may be longer, stronger or closer together - but not all three. False labor will always stop when you change your activity or shift position, or drink fluids (dehydration can cause false labor contractions).

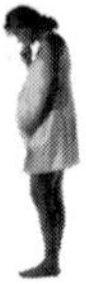

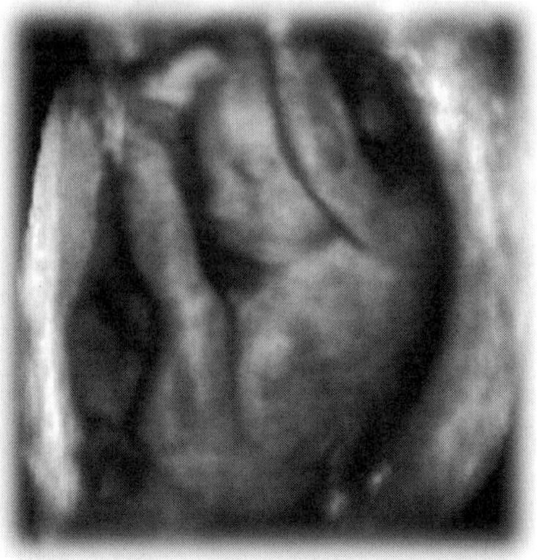

DAY 210

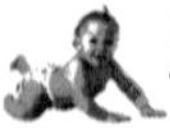

Babies can swim. Not just in amniotic fluid but in water. The swimming reflex - head down, arms and legs flailing, exhaling slowing through the mouth - is present now. Realtime ultrasound studies of babies shows that they smile ten times more often now at 30 weeks than they will at birth. The pupillary light reflex - the pupil constricting in response to bright light - is present.

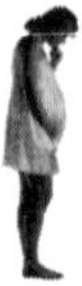

True labor contractions: The entire uterus hardens. The contractions do follow a pattern; becoming regular and stronger. They do get longer, stronger and closer together. Finally, they don't stop when you move or change position. In fact, walking around may make them even stronger.

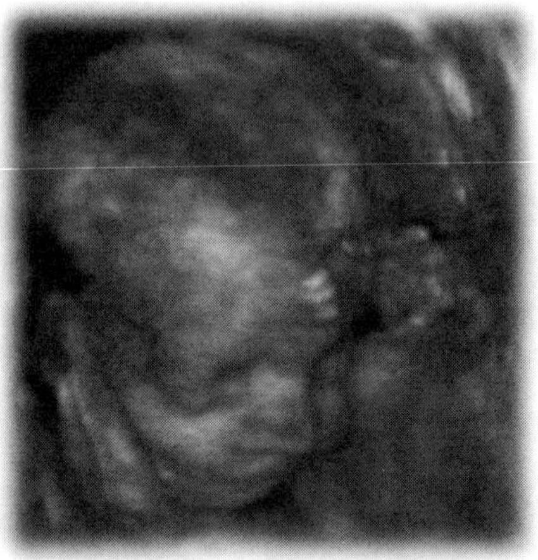

Thoughts:

....

....

DAY 211

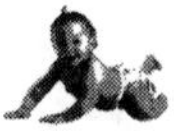

The chemical senses of your baby (taste and smell) have been functioning since the 12th week and your baby has acquired lots of information. It has learned about the food you eat by transfer of chemical molecules through the blood. It has learned your odors as well. Newborns prefer to nurse from their mother's breast rather than that of another lactating female. This preference can be eliminated by wiping odors from the mother's lactating breast onto another woman's breast. Babies learn about these chemical stimuli from agents in the mother's blood *in utero* and seek them out. Furthermore, bottle-fed babies which have had no direct experience with nursing at their mother's breast, still prefer the mother's breast odors compared to another female's. Baby is 19.5 inches ❦ 4-1/2 lbs.

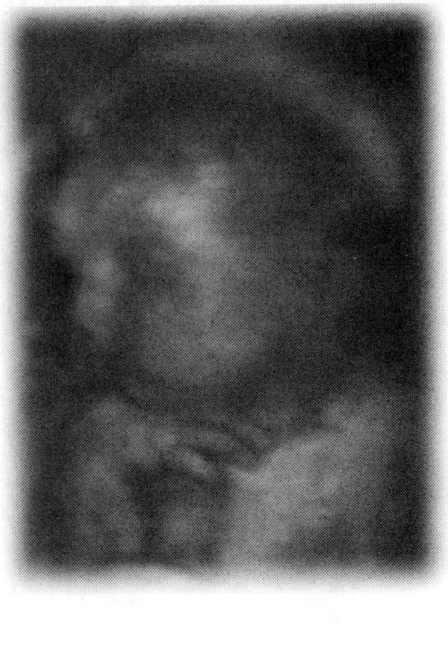

Notes:

....

....

DAY 212

Your baby's eyes are open and the visual system is working, although there isn't much to look at. Babies can perceive all sorts of things that we take for granted. One is biological motion. This is the awareness that something that's moving is alive. Infants prefer to look at the patterns produced by luminous dots on the elbows, knees, legs, torso and arms of a human jogging in place compared to the patterns produced by the random movement of dots. This suggest that there is an innate, hardwired mechanism directing visual attention to potentially meaningful events (people or animals moving nearby).

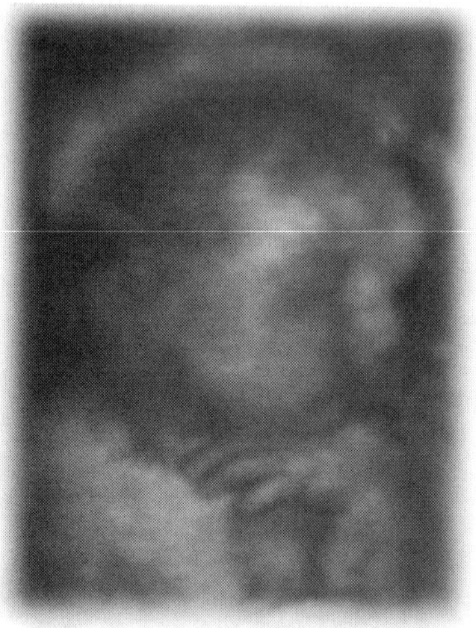

Thoughts:

....

....

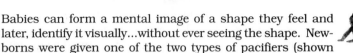

Babies can form a mental image of a shape they feel and later, identify it visually...without ever seeing the shape. Newborns were given one of the two types of pacifiers (shown below) to suck on. The pacifiers were placed into and removed from the babies mouths without the baby seeing the nipple. Babies who sucked on the nobby nipple looked longer at it than the smooth nipple; while babies that sucked on the smooth nipple looked longer at it. This experiment demonstrates that babies can form an internal representation (a memory) in one sensory modality (touch) and use it to identify the object in another sense (vision). Scientists call this ability cross-modal matching. For adults this is similar to reaching blindly into the back of a cluttered drawer searching for a key. We have a mental representation of the key - discarding mismatches along the way - when we locate what feels like a key we pull it out of the drawer. Babies have similar abilities that can be demonstrated when they are asked in a way that conforms to their abilities.

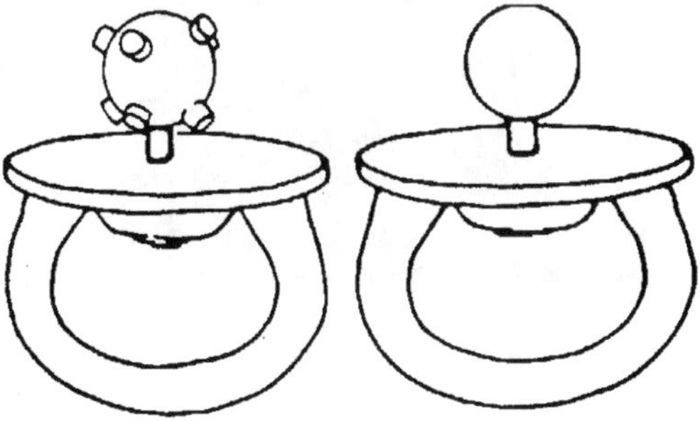

from Meltzoff & Borton (1979).

DAY 214

Some mothers have higher heart rates than others. Two groups were formed based on resting maternal heart rate at 31 weeks. One group of babies had mothers with heart rates of 70-80 beats per minute; another group with mothers' heart rates between 100-110 beats/minute (designated as the high heart rate group). Two days after birth, the babies born to the low heart rate mothers fell asleep faster, slept longer and cried less, compared to babies born to mothers in the high heart rate group. Are you likely to have an "easy" baby? Check your crystal ball by determining your resting heart rate (take your wrist pulse count the number of beats in a 15 second period and multiply by 4.)

Baby holding her hand out

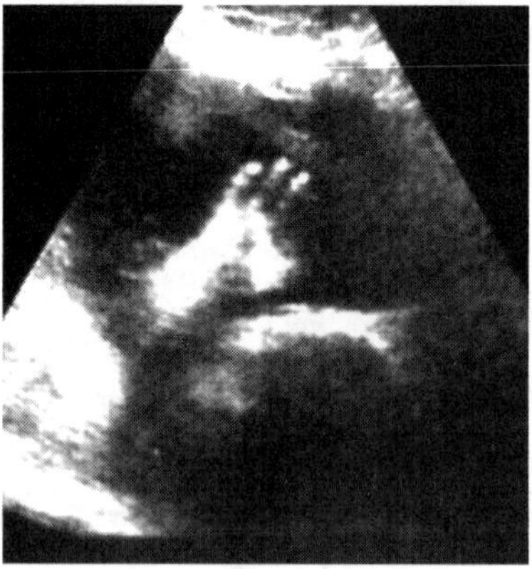

Thoughts:

....

....

DAY 215

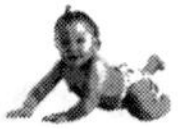

Your baby has been swallowing amniotic fluid for quite some time now. The tongue movements that accompany swallowing have been shown to play an important role in forming the shape of the top of the mouth (the palate). In animal studies where the normal movements of the tongue has been blocked, malformed palates have resulted.

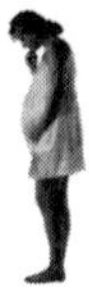

During your last 30 days of pregnancy, estrogen production will increase. This will enhance muscle contractions, softening of the cervix and effacement, and will promote blood clotting. Oxytocin receptors also increase in uterine and abdominal muscle. When oxytocin is applied to these receptors, the strong, and significantly different. muscle contractions of labor occur.

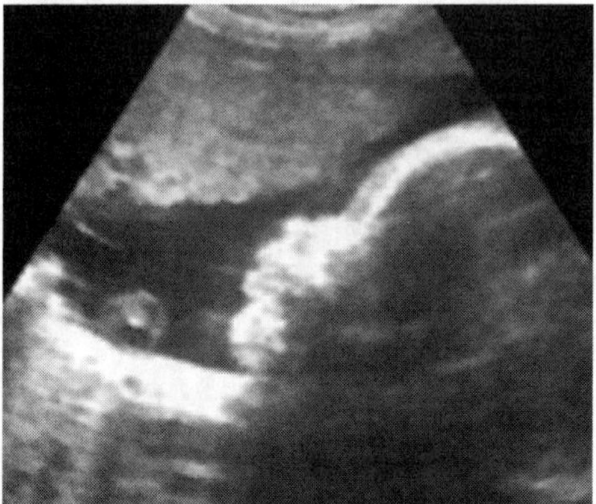

Notes:

....

....

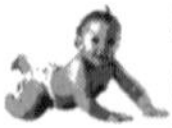

Sucking on a nipple is a task that babies can easily perform. Babies will suck more during something they like. Sucking can be used to ask babies what they prefer, and what they can learn and remember. Babies can learn to suck to produce their mother's voice, and prefer their mother's voice over that of another woman. The more the sound of the voice matches what the babies are accustomed to hearing, the more they like it. Babies prefer a version of their mother's voice that is modified to sound like it would *in utero* complete with background heart beats, indicating that the baby learns and remembers what's going on in the womb. Interestingly, by three weeks after birth, the baby prefers the mother's unfiltered, normal voice. After all your voice transmitted through the air is now what your baby is familiar with.

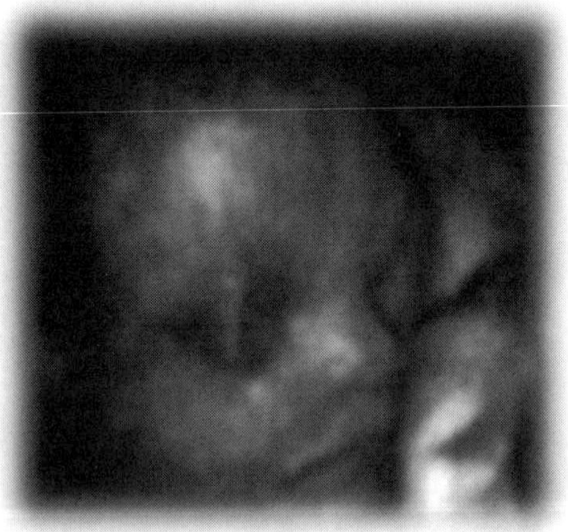

Thoughts

....

....

DAY 217

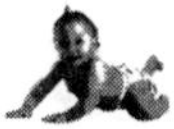

Your baby's eyes will be open when she's not sleeping. All babies usually have blue eyes until a few weeks after birth. Exposure to light cause the pigments to change into their genetically programmed final colors.

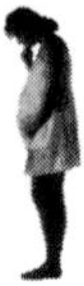

With all the changes in your body during pregnancy there are a number of conditions that can lead to fainting. Extremely hot weather, standing for too long a time, standing in a crowd and standing up too fast all can make you feel light-headed and you could faint.

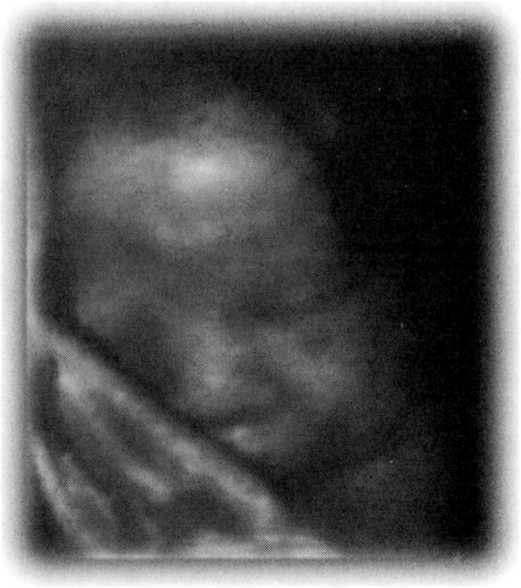

Notes:

....

....

Are babies paying attention to the language being spoken...do they care if you're speaking English or Spanish? Using the preferential sucking test, scientists have asked this question. Babies prefer what is familiar. Babies suck more during spoken English if their mother speaks English. If their English-speaking mother speaks Spanish the babies show no preference for the mother's voice over another woman's. Babies attend to the intonation and sounds of a language more than they do to the speaker...in this case, the mother.

Baby is 20 inches ❦ 5.0 lbs.

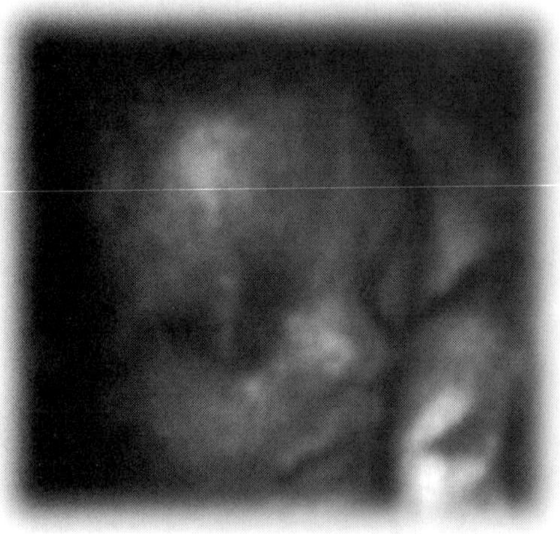

Thoughts:

....

....

DAY 219

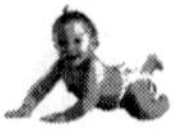

Your baby will respond with a brief increase in activity to a vibrating stimulus (essentially an electric toothbrush touched to your abdomen). The baby will habituate (grow accustomed) to the stimulus and won't respond after about 10 applications of the stimulus. There is a sex difference with girl babies responding sooner - at about 25 weeks - while boys respond later, at about 28 weeks.

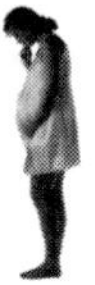

Many women experience foot pain due to the increased weight they're carrying, center of gravity shifts and fluid retention. The best way to prevent foot problems is by wearing shoes that have good arch support. Put your feet up to relieve swelling, avoid foods high in sodium to alleviate fluid retention and take frequent walks to keep your blood circulating.

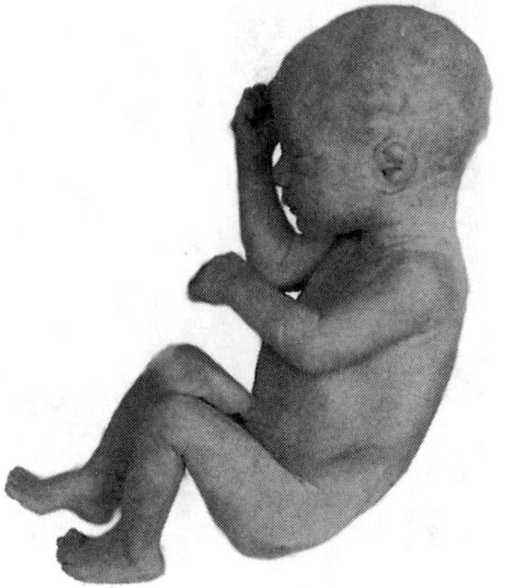

Notes:

....

....

The rate of habituation of this movement response to the vibrating stimulus, just like the visual attention response discussed earlier, is also predictive of later intelligence measured at birth, 4 months and 1 yr. Normal fetal movement habituation was associated with better scores on the Brazelton Scale taken right at birth. At 4 months of age, faster habituators had significantly higher mental development scores on the Bayley Scales of Infant Development. And fetuses who habituated faster showed higher scores on a Mental Development Scale at 1 yr of age.

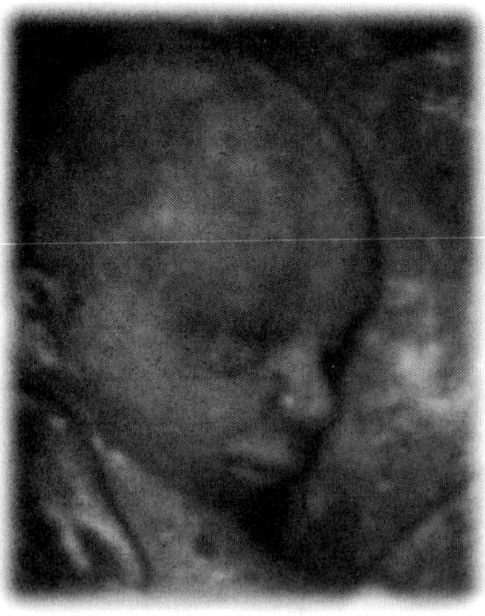

Thoughts:

....

....

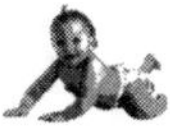

Babies spend about 80% of their time in rapid eye movement (REM) sleep. Brain development occurs during REM sleep as cerebral metabolism, blood flow and protein synthesis all greatly increase. Protein synthesis occurs when new structure (neurons and supporting structures) are being manufactured and sculpted.

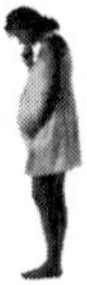

The cervix is usually capped by a 'mucous plug' that prevents fluid from entering the uterus. The mucous plug can become dislodged at any point during the pregnancy, and will reform. Because the plug can come loose anytime it is not a reliable predictor of the onset of labor.

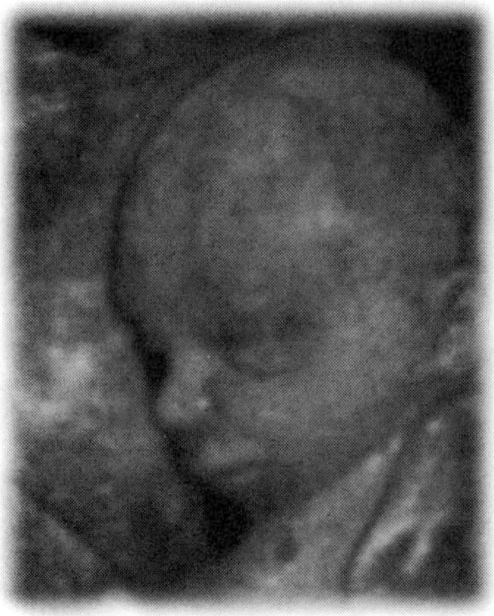

Notes:

....

....

DAY 222

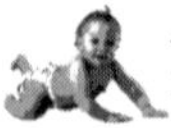

A very small percentage of babies are born before their bodies are ready for the transition to the outside world. Modern medicine has made a number of advances to help ensure the survival of premature babies. One is the administration of steroid hormones. Giving steroid hormones to the mother will dramatically accelerate the maturation of the baby's vital organs. The hormonal treatment is effective even if given only 24 hours before birth.

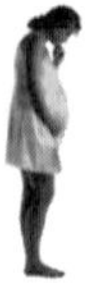

Many of the treatments that are effective in helping prematurely-born babies are similar to naturally occurring events in the womb. One is the finding that massage and handling of a premature baby facilitates its progress and development. The constant activity inside the womb from mother-generated movements like walking and Braxton-Hicks contractions provide lots of tactile stimulation for the baby.

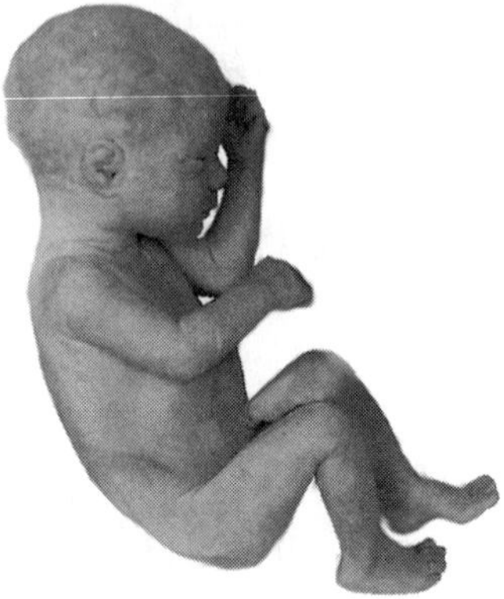

Thoughts:

....

....

DAY 223

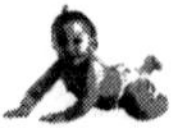

One of the major features that apparently is unique to great apes, including humans, is a sense of self: A demonstrable appreciation that we are separate and distinct from others, unique, with free will. Self-concept or self-awareness is difficult to demonstrate in non-speaking infants. One test - called the rouge test - involves a spot of red rouge makeup being placed on the baby's forehead (without the baby seeing it placed there) and then exposing the baby to a mirror. Noticing the spot and trying to touch it is taken as evidence that A: the baby notices the spot as different; and B: that the spot is not consistent with the image of self that the baby is familiar with. To demonstrate self-concept with this test requires fine motor control (to point) and visual skills that may be beyond the baby's capabilities. No wonder self-concept 'appears' at 18 months of age using this test.

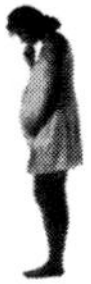

Oxytocin (Pitocin®) is a hormone that can facilitate and speed up labor. If contractions stall, oxytocin can restart uterine activity and contractions. Oxytocin also assists in the contraction of the distended uterus after birth.

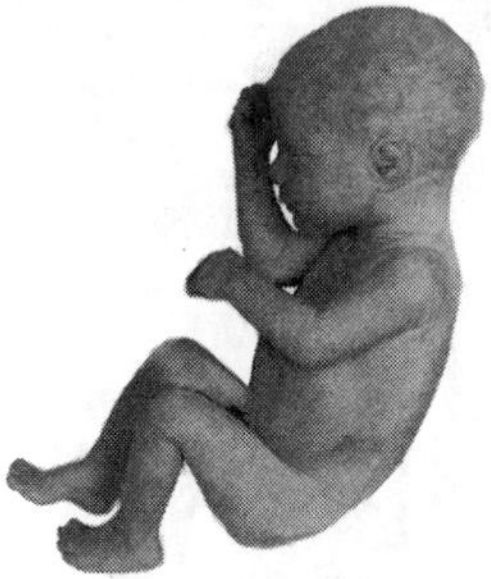

Notes:

....

....

Babies are great imitators. In fact, they are born imitators and learn by imitation. Newborns have the fascinating ability to reproduce or imitate facial expressions they see performed by someone else. This ability requires the operation and coordination of many complex processes. The baby must take in the visual information it sees, process those cues and generate a pattern of muscular contractions which recreate the image it sees, to describe just a few of the processes involved. Quite a feat.

The top series of photos shows a adult making a variety of facial expressions. Below is the baby's imitative facial response.

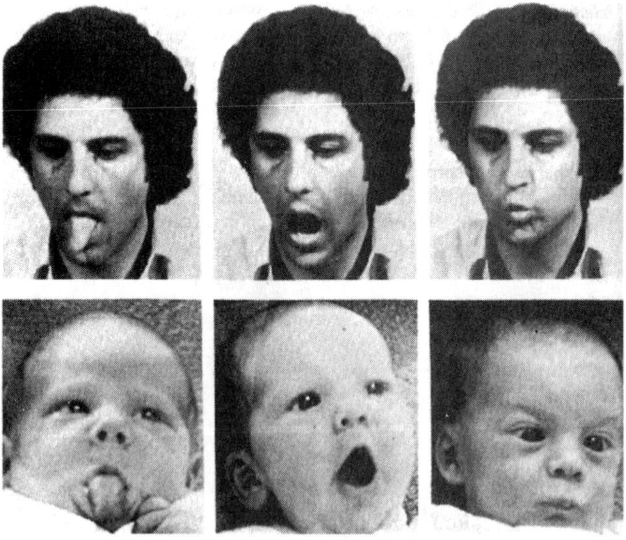

from Meltzoff & Moore (1977).

DAY 225

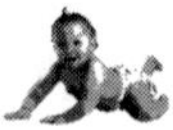

Today starts the 9th month of your pregnancy. Your baby is ready to go, and will put on some additional weight as birth approaches.

Baby is 20 inches ❦ 5-1/2 lbs.

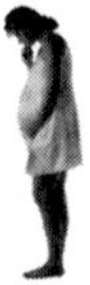

About now you'll probably have your prenatal visits weekly. In addition to taking your weight, blood pressure, measuring the size of the baby and urine test, your cervix may be examined to see if effacement has started and you'll be asked about the frequency of your Braxton-Hicks contractions.

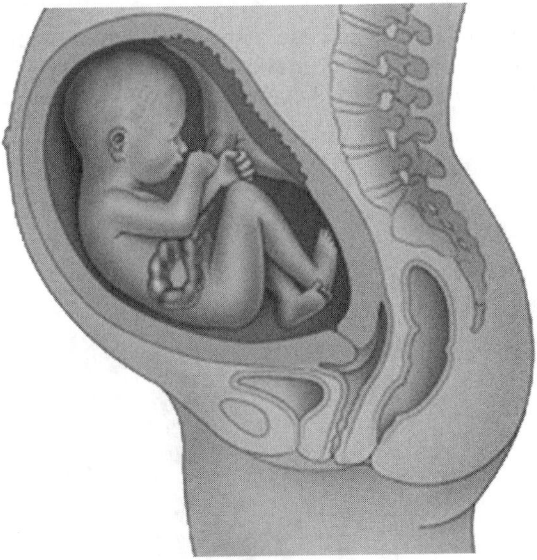

Notes:

Neurophysiological studies with monkeys have shown that simply watching another monkey perform a simple motor task causes the neurons in the observing monkey's brain to fire as if the observing monkey were actually performing the movement. This suggests that an infant observing a facial expression has a 'priming' neural discharge that 'coaches' the neurons to fire in such a manner to produce the facial response. No practice, just performance. Imitation provides an initial basis for the development of social bonds between baby and caretaker. Parents love babies to imitate their behavior and babies love when parents imitate what they are doing.

The umbilical cord is coated by a gel-like substance that inhibits bleeding when the cord is cut. No pain will be felt by either you or your baby because there are no pain receptors in the cord.

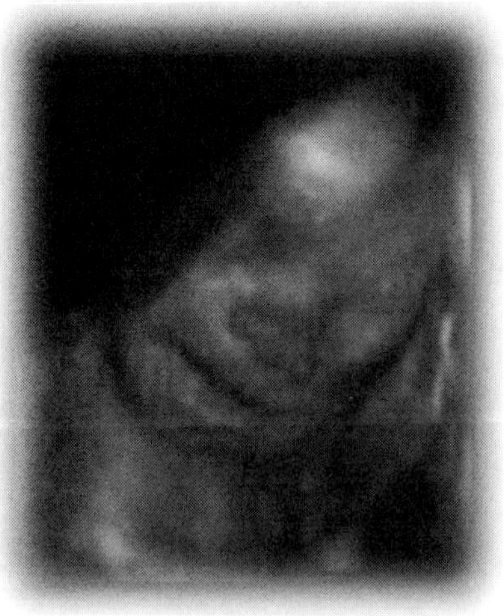

DAY 227

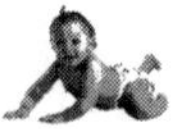

If imitation serves to foster social ties, then babies should prefer adults who imitate them too. In the following study a subject baby sat in an infant seat across a table from two adults. One of the adults matched everything the baby did; the other adult matched the behavior of another baby (out of view of the test baby). Both adults acted like babys, however only one of the adults imitated the subject baby. Babies directed more visual attention (in the form of looking longer) and smiled more at the person who was imitating them. They showed a clear preference for the adult that was imitating them.

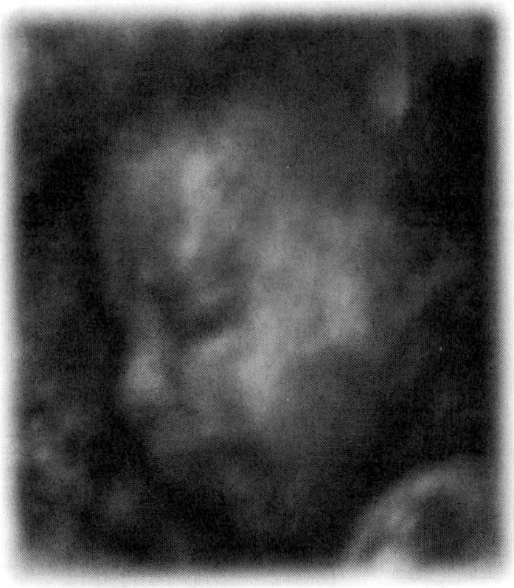

Notes:

....

....

Motherese - the high pitched, sing-song voice mothers use when talking to their babies is another example of imitation. Both mother and child imitate each other. Shown below is a voice print of the mother and baby as they imitate each other's voice in an amazing 'conversation' of pitch and frequencies of sound. Infants love to be imitated - as you'll see from the squeals of delight that they show during the game.

Shown is a "voice-print" record of the interaction between mother and daughter. The mother says the phrases indicated below the record and the baby responds after (d) with sounds that match the mother's.

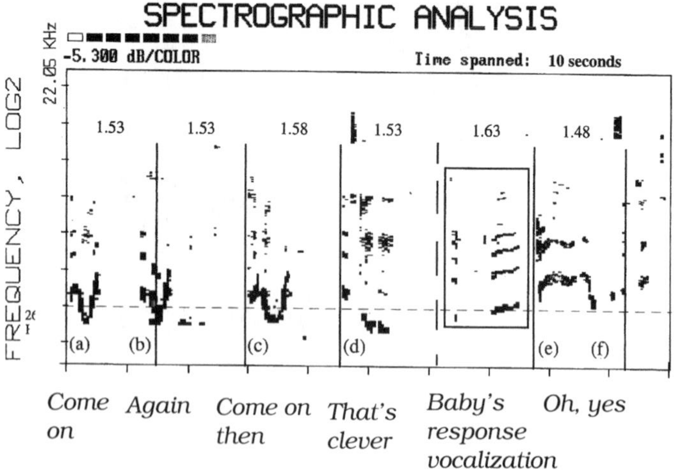

from Trevarthan et al., 1999

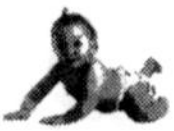

Babies this age are sleeping most of the time. How much information from the environment can the baby get if it's asleep? Babies are very attentive and responsive to outside stimulation while they sleep. Stable heart rate is a characteristic of quiet sleep. When you speak your baby shows a decrease in heart rate - which indicates it's paying attention and listening to your speech. If you were to just whisper (create the same breathing movements but the sound is too weak to hear) your baby doesn't show any heart rate attentional response because it didn't hear your voice. Babies aren't using sleep to tune out - they are attentive information processors during sleep.

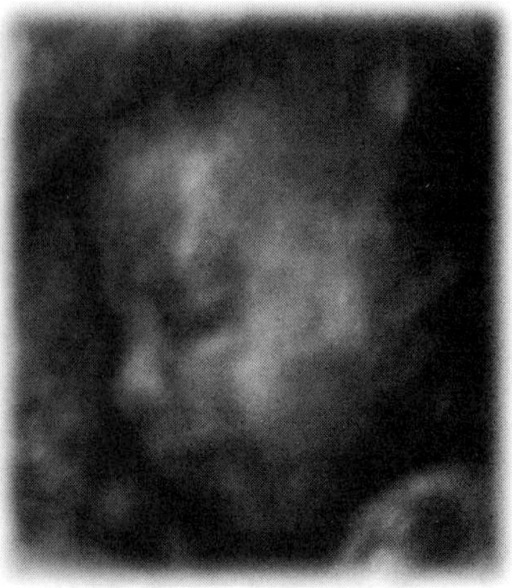

Notes:

....

....

DAY 230

There is a invariant sequence in the onset and development of the senses. The order of appearance is Tactile ➜ Vestibular ➜ Chemical (Taste/Smell) ➜ Auditory ➜ Visual. This order of appearance is important for the normal functioning of these sensory systems. Presenting chicks with early visual stimulation (by removing the top half of their shell and presenting a few brief light pulses) disrupted their normal response to auditory cues (maternal calls) from the hen. Essentially these chicks didn't come when called by the hen after hatching, as do normal chicks. The timing of stimulation is important for the normal development of the brain and the expression of behavior.

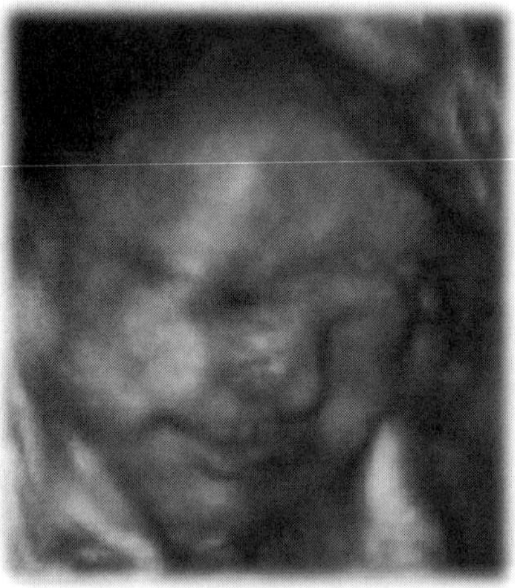

Thoughts:

....

....

DAY 231

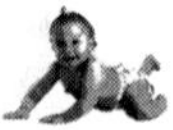

The relative absence of visual stimulation in the womb may help fetal sensory systems develop without competition or interference. For example, given the dominance of the visual system, 'mis-timed' early exposure to visual stimuli could result in visual brain areas colonizing other brain areas earmarked for auditory function. Attempts to fool with Mother Nature by presenting unnatural or too much stimulation to the fetus, as could occur with so-called *Prenatal Universities*, may do more harm than good.

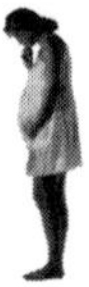

Breast milk is composed of protein, carbohydrates and fats. Most of the foods that you eat don't affect the taste or composition of breast milk, but some substances can transfer into breast milk and be passed to the baby. Almost all over-the-counter drugs like aspirin and caffeine and alcohol, most prescription drugs, pesticides, strong tasting spices like garlic, and laxatives get to your baby through breast milk.

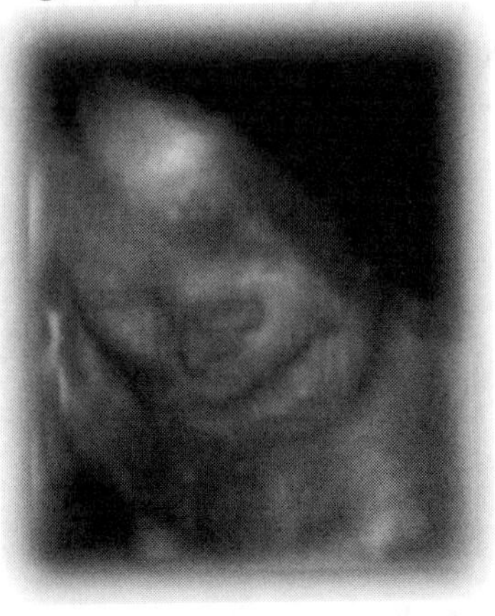

Notes:

....

....

Why do babies have such fat cheeks? There are at least two scientific reasons. The first is that the extra thickness of the cheeks prevent them from collapsing while sucking - helpful if you're going to rely on sucking for nutrients. Second is that fat cheeks and a round head contribute to the perception of 'cuteness' by adults of infant animals, including human babies - helpful in encouraging parental nuturance, along with a smile or two.

Baby is 20.5 inches ❦ 6.0 lbs.

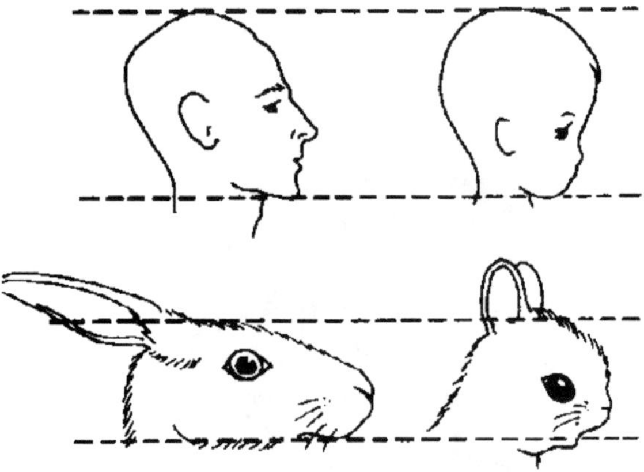

from Alley (1981).

Thoughts:

....

....

DAY 233

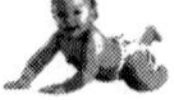

Babies are made to learn. They learn about their environment through their senses and they learn about social interactions through imitation. Place a baby in an infant carrier in a room, turn out the lights and she will first look around, then reach out and search for stimulation, for information. Babies are biologically programmed to seek novel or new information.

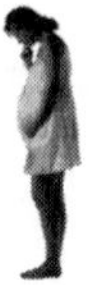

Regular bathing is important and will not have any adverse effects on the baby. Be sure not to have the water too hot as you could become dizzy. Bathing will not result in dirty water entering the uterus and infecting the baby.

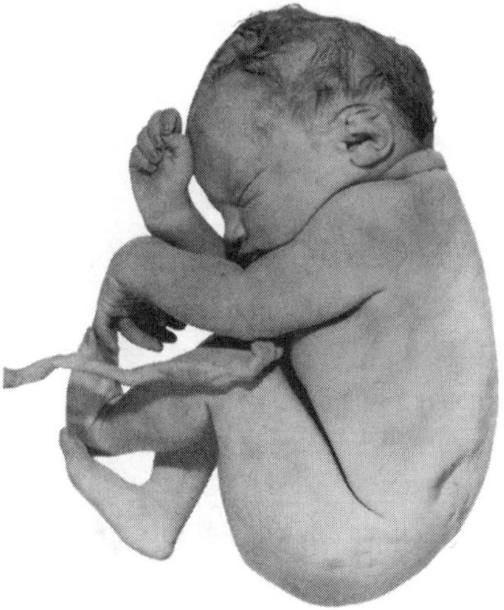

Notes:

....

....

DAY 234

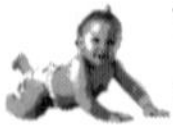

What does the word mind mean to you? Philosophers and scientists have considered various definitions and what constitutes evidence of mind for many years. One definition is the awareness that one is separate and distinct from others - a sense of self or self-concept. Unfortunately we can't ask babies to speak to us and tell us 'who they are' or ask them to reliably perform complex motor tasks - like the rouge test - to prove what they know.

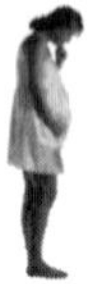

Your pelvic joints may feel different due to the slight relaxation of the periarticular structures, including a slight widening of the joint space of the pubic bone. Mother Nature is preparing your body for birth.

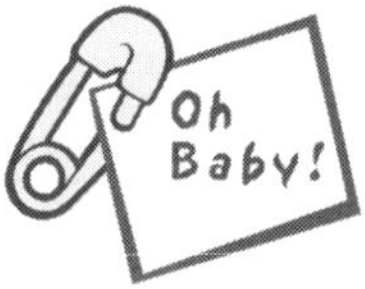

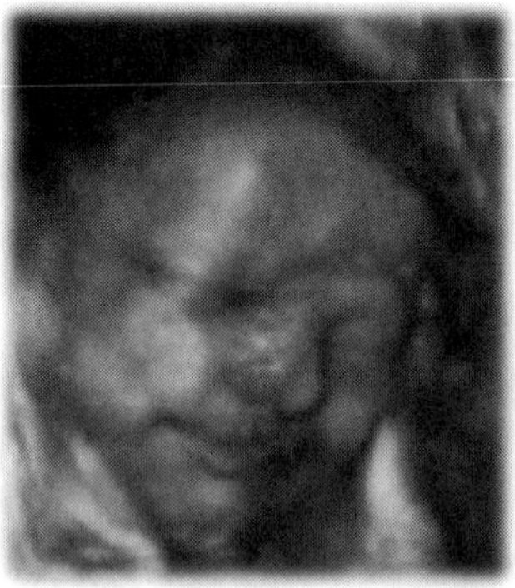

Thoughts:

....

....

DAY 235

Human newborns, unlike other animals, may be born with an innate sense of self. Using a simple habituation test two-week old babies were shown a variety of slides of baby faces on a screen - all types of babies. After seeing 10 or 15 slides of baby faces, the infant gets bored and looks less and less at each subsequent slide. However, when shown a picture of him or herself - the babies looked a long time at the photo. It appeared that babies habituated to the initial series of photos because, while all the photos were different, they were the same in one respect - they were all photos of *other* babies. When the baby saw himself on screen he looked longer because he noticed something different. *That's me!* is what the baby's behavior suggested. This elegantly simple experiment suggested that 2 week old babies recognize themselves as different from other babies and perhaps have a sense of self.

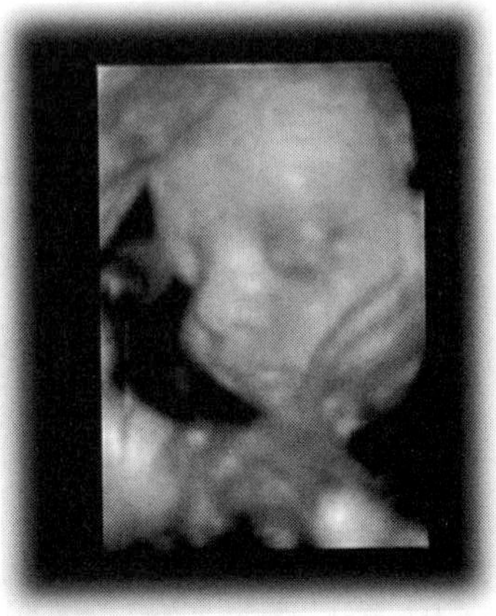

Notes:

....

....

DAY 236

What colors can your baby see? Babies can see the same spectrum of color that we can. This has been tested using an habituation procedure. Presentation of the same color over and over predicatbly causes the baby to look less and less, change the color, and the baby looks longer. The baby tells us from the increased looking or attentional response that they notice and can see the change. This is how we know that babies can see color.

Your labor may be similar to your mother or sister's labor experiences. Since there are similar genetic makeups and corresponding anatomy between close relatives, there can be a relationship. For example, thick, dense pelvic musculature could lead to longer labor because more stretching and relaxation must occur to get the baby through the birth canal. Also, the size of the pelvic opening (os) is a key factor in the ease of labor and delivery, as well as the baby's size and the position of its head while moving through the pelvic os.

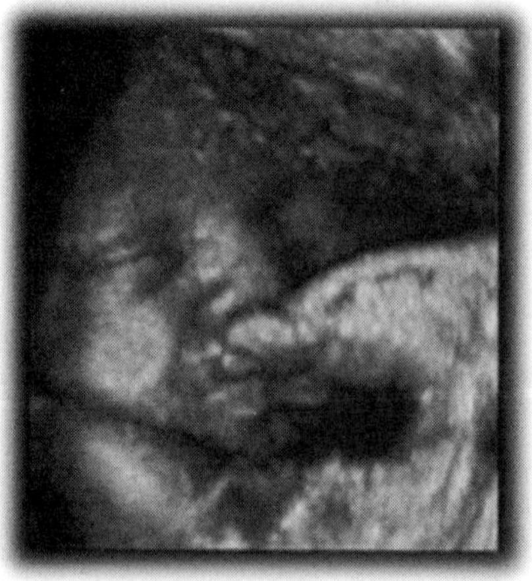

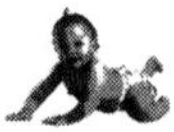

Colors exist along a continuum. There are lots of shades of blue that melt into shades of green. Light is a physical thing measured by its wavelength. Blue light is a wavelength around 450 nanometers (billionths of a meter); green is 530 nm and yellow is 600 nm. Adults report that lights of 450 nm and 480 nm are different shades of blue. Experiments with babies have shown that they recognize shades of color, (using the habituation technique to demonstrate recognition of a new shade). Babies see shades of blue as blue, categorically distinct from green, just like adults do. So your baby will notice whether his sleeper is baby blue or teal...whether he really cares what color it is another story entirely.

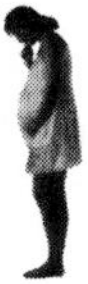

Fatigue during the 9th month is common, as most women find it difficult to sleep at night. Pressure against the diaphragm from the enlarged uterus can cause acid reflux, or heart burn, when lying down. Try sleeping in a reclined position with several pillows to elevate your head and keep the acid down. Be sure to check with your doctor before taking any over-the-counter heartburn remedies.

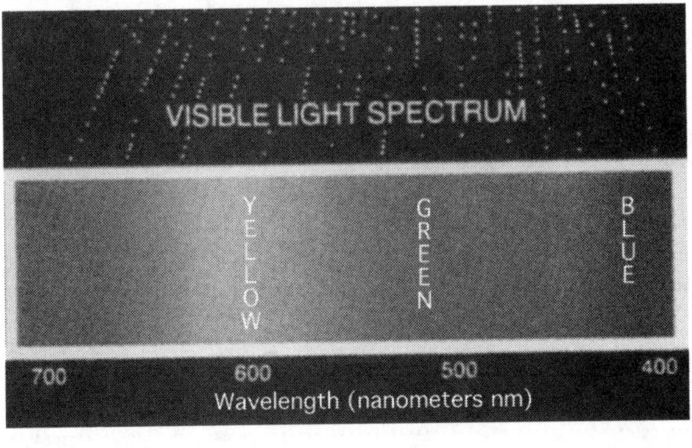

DAY 238

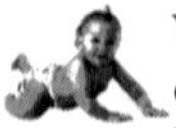

Your baby can localize sound. Babies can determine which direction a sound is coming from just like an adult. Sound localization is accomplished in the brain by computing the slight difference in time of the arrival of the sound waves at each ear. In the diagram below, sound waves reach the left ear earlier, causing a head turn to the left. Babies, if supported in a special baby hammock, will turn their heads left or right to correctly locate the source of a sound.

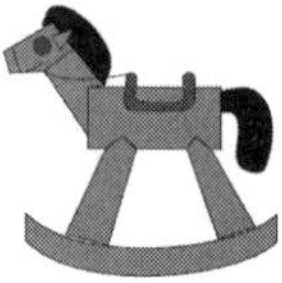

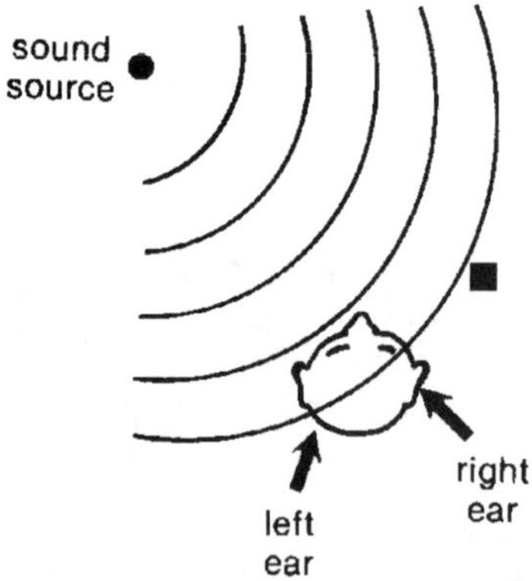

Thoughts:

....

....

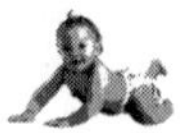

Basic neurophysiological research has shown that a baby's brain responds to the visual characteristics of color and brightness, and also to more complex features as well such as edges, contours and movement of light across the eye. These feature detector neurons, as they are called, indicate that the fetal brain has an innate capability for complex form and depth perception. For example, babies prefer to look at faces vs. unpatterned grayscale images. Faces are composed of forms, edges and contours that activate the brain's visual feature detectors. So the next time someone says they find you beautiful tell them you really know they are just interested in your forms and contours.

Baby is 21 inches ❦ 6.5 lbs.

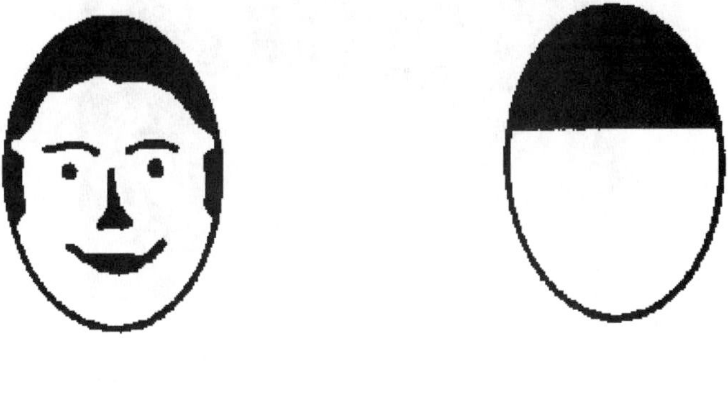

Babies prefer to look at faces compared to stimuli with less forms and contours.

from Fantz (1963)

DAY 240

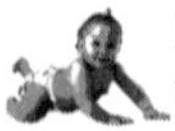

How well can a baby see? Until 1960 or so, many thought that babies were born functionally blind, that they really couldn't see in any meaningful or functional way. In fact, a baby's visual system is set up now to focus clearly on objects that are 8 -10 inches away. They see as well as adults at this distance. And when you hold your baby in your arms guess how far her face is from yours...8 - 10 inches!

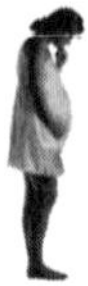

Labor duration - First-time mothers should expect to be in labor for 12 - 24 hours. Only 5% of all first babies arrive in fewer than 5 hours. For second-time or more moms, labor is usually about half the time of the first baby.

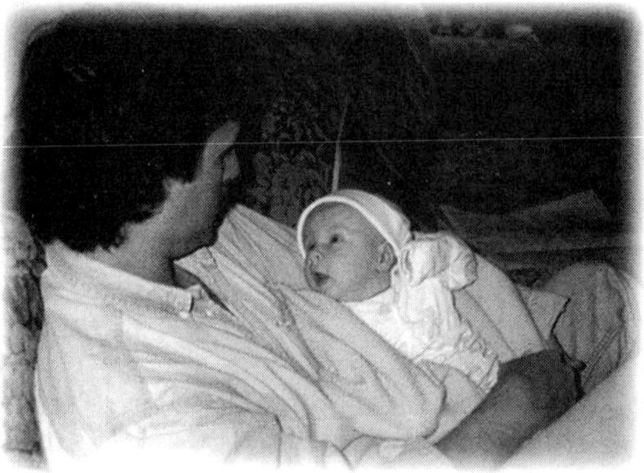

Thoughts:

....

....

DAY 241

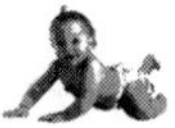

We see circles and squares are complete things, not a constellation of the individual lines and angles that form them. Do babies see shapes as we do? A very clever test using figures that generate visual illusions, known as subjective contours, was used to answer this question. The figure on the left contains a square (which is an illusion) that is formed as a result of the alignment of the four circular segments...see it? The figure on the right does not contain the illusion because the elements are misaligned. Babies were shown one figure until they habituated (looked less and less); then shown the other figure. Babies shown the figure with the square illusion habituated to the illusion, and then looked more (dishabituated) when the illusion was gone, that is, when the figure was changed. Babies do see forms as integrated wholes just as we do; not just collages of the elements (lines, angles) that make up the forms.

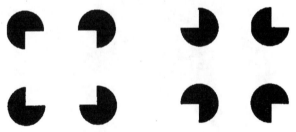

Figure containing square illusion

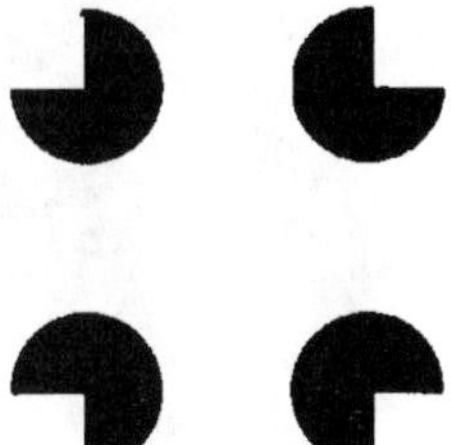

No illusion, just the elements

from Bertenthal, Campos & Haith (1980).

Notes:

....

....

DAY 242

Your baby's lungs are probably mature and ready to go. Surfactant - a detergent-like molecule - that prevents the alveoli (air sacs) in the lung from sticking together on exhaling is present, enabling normal inspiration and expiration. In babies born very early, artificial surfactant has been developed that greatly enhances lung function. Also other drugs have been developed that can increase oxygen absorption into the blood, which has the effect of enhancing oxygenation of the blood. Because of advances like these, prematurely born babies have a much greater chance of survival than they did just a decade ago.

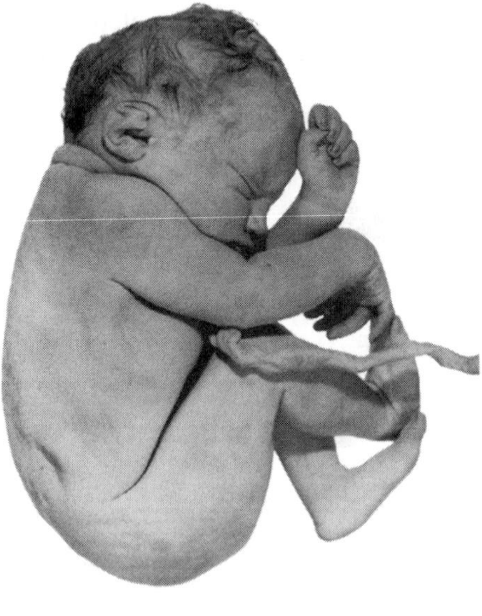

Thoughts:

....

....

DAY 243

Facial expressions are innate, hardwired patterns of muscular activation that signal emotional state. These expressions are universally recognized for their meaning. A smile, a frown, a sad face are recognized similarly for what they mean across all cultures, even isolated cultures with little or no outside contact with others. Babies communicate their emotional state as well. Smiling by a baby means 'I like this, let's keep doing this.' Crying is a signal that something is wrong and must be changed. There are even different sound fingerprints (complete with a different facial expression) for different cries that signal hunger vs. anger. vs. pain. Facial expressions transmit information to the outside world about the baby's emotional state. Both smiling and crying bring caregivers near, thereby enhancing the baby's chances of survival.

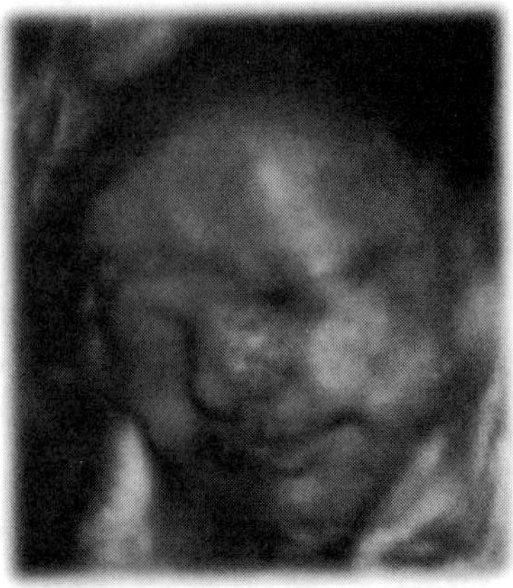

Notes:

....

....

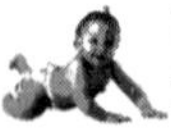

Babies can 'read' the difference between different facial expressions. For example, they can see the difference between a facial expression of happiness vs. one of fear or anger. In an experiment babies were shown a series of faces that contained a happy facial expression. The faces were all of different people, but they were similar in that they were all smiling - showing a happy face. Eventually the babies get bored with the smiling faces and look less & less (habituate). Then they are shown the test face (one depicting another emotion like surprise or anger). The babies dishabituate and look longer. This increase in visual attention indicates that the baby noticed something different: the change in emotional state represented by the facial expression. If angry expressions are shown first, then a happy face later, the baby shows the same dishabituation response, again indicating that they learn the emotion represented by the face and pay attention when the facial expression shown changes.

Happy training stimuli

Happy, surprise & anger test faces

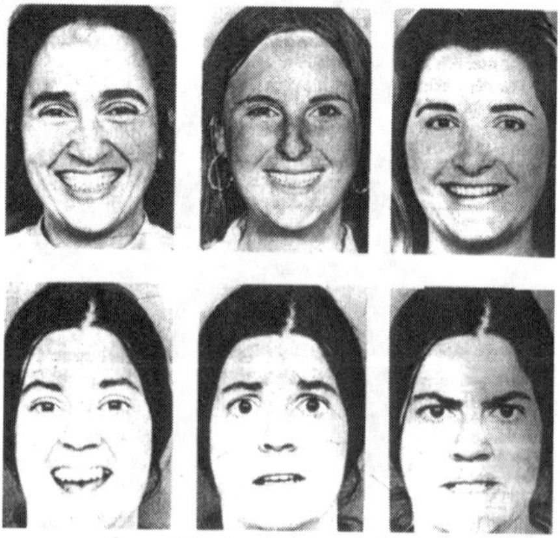

from Kestenbaum & Nelson (1990).

DAY 245

Babies prefer attractive faces. Just like adults, babies prefer to look at attractive faces compared to unattractive faces. To test this, a set of photographs was produced that was divided into attractive and unattractive groupings based on rating by adults (the faces were of all types: infants, adults, male, female, white, black). Then babies were shown an attractive and an unattractive face side by side. The experimenters simply measured how long the baby looked at each. Babies looked twice as long at the attractive face compared to the unattractive face . With adults as subjects, it could easily be argued that the key features that are perceived as attractive are learned from experience - images seen in magazines and on television. However, these experiments with babies show that facial attractiveness is actually innate, not learned.

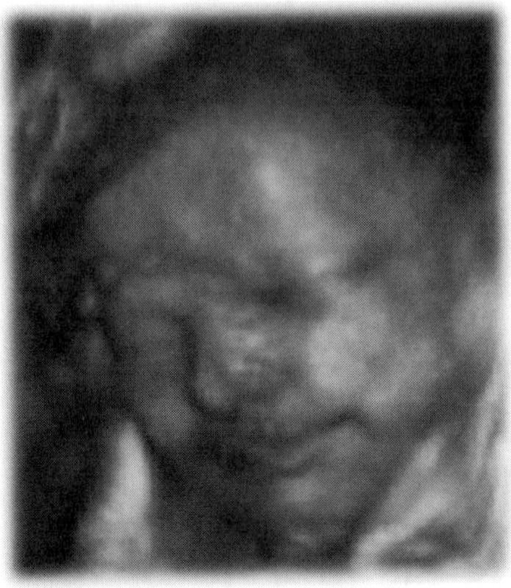

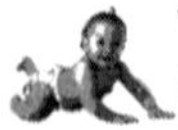

What makes for an attractive face? Scientists have shown that when faces are computer-averaged that the resulting prototype is typically seen as more attractive than any of the individual faces from which the prototype was formed. Attractive faces may be perceived as more 'face-like' therefore they are preferred.

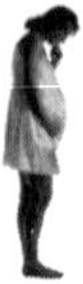

Your doctor or midwife will probably examine your cervix for signs of dilation as well as effacement, or softening. If you've been having erratic contractions, or 'false labor', these mini-contractions may have caused some changes in your cervix. When your cervix is measured, its size is estimated using the pinky or forefinger, and will be given in centimeters. A cervix dilated 1 centimeter would be open this much.

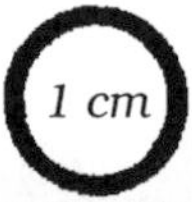

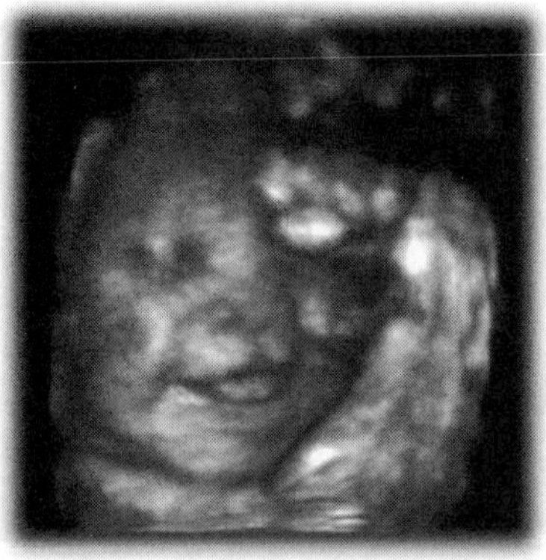

Thoughts: Baby is 22 inches ❦ 6.8 lbs.

....

....

DAY 247

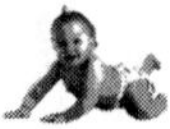

Can babies feel pain? In rare medical conditions that require fetal blood transfusions, measurements of hormones associated with pain and stress increase. Internal opioids like beta endorphin increase five-fold; cortisol, a stress hormone, increases almost two-fold. In studies with adults, a correlation has been established with these opioid levels increasing as the perceived pain and stress levels increased. It is, therefore, reasonable to conclude that babies feel pain as we do.

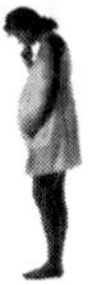

If you give birth to a boy and you're considering circumcision there is no reason not to use topical, local anesthetic. The myth that babies don't feel pain - repeated by anyone whom you view as a medical professional - should prompt you to question their training and expertise.

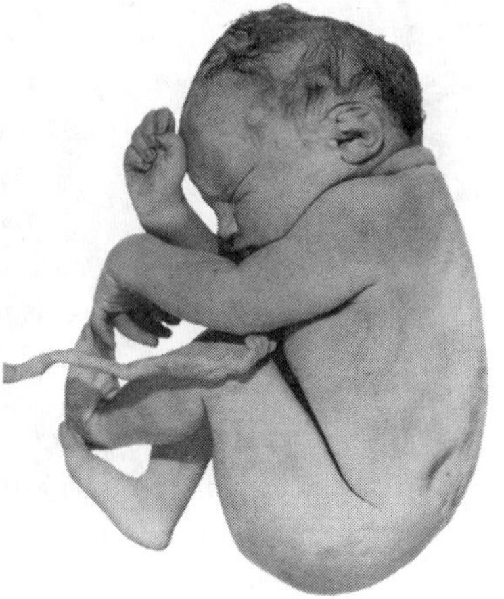

Notes:

....

....

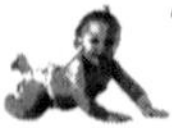

There are a variety of physiological measures associated with emotional state, one of which is sweating. When we become anxious, concerned or in pain, we sweat. Babies subject to a blood drawing procedure (heel-prick) showed emotionally-induced sweating at 29 weeks.

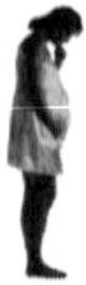

You should have your hospital bags packed and ready to go just in case you're early. Have a plan of action prepared so you'll be able to stay calm and get to the hospital.

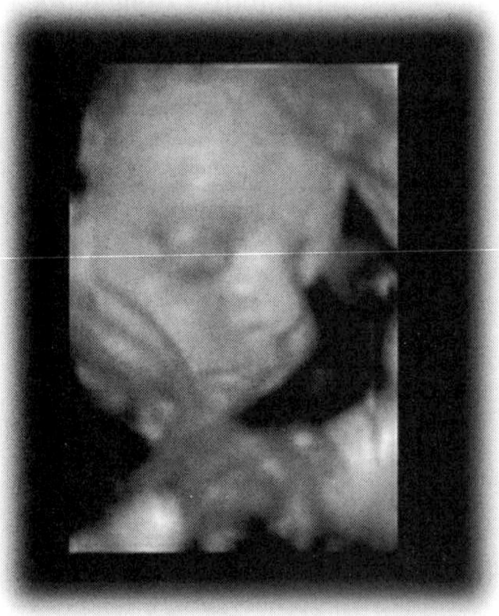

Thoughts:

....

....

DAY 249

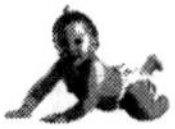

We know that a photograph is just a two-dimensional representation of a real person. We recognize a person from their photo. Babies can do the same. Using a preferential looking test, babies were shown a photograph of a person (they hadn't seen before) until they got bored. The test was to have two people stand side-by-side in front of the baby - one person from the photograph, the other a stranger. The babies preferred to look at the stranger because they had gotten bored looking at the person in the photo. This shows that babies can transfer a representation of a person, as in a photo, from 2 dimensions to 3, and retain the image in memory for use later.

*** An important distinction with respect to preferential looking to keep in mind is this: In general, if the image has no emotional significance, babies prefer novel images (as they did above). When the image has emotional significance (like the mother's face or voice) babies prefer the familiar.***

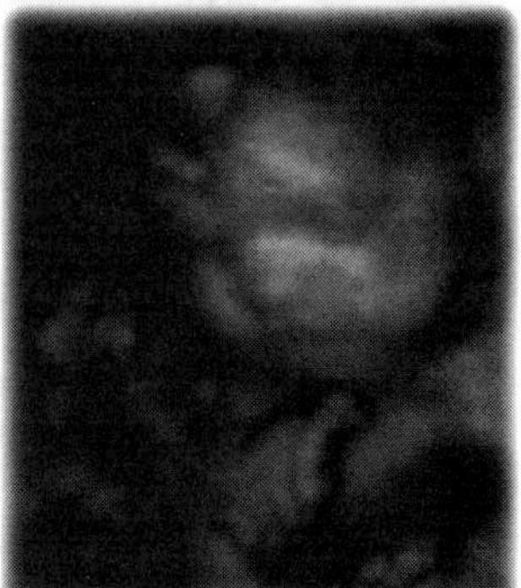

Notes:

....

....

DAY 250

Boy babies and girl babies have different body temperatures. A study of 105 babies found that core body temperature was significantly higher in girls (37.168° C / 98.902°F) than boys (37.068°C / 98.722°F). Now we know the explanation of why teenage boys want to be 'cool' and teenage girls want to be seen as 'hot': they're born that way! There are several metabolic differences between boy and girl babies. Newborn female babies have more body fat mass than do males. Part of that fat is in the form of brown fat tissue which is involved in thermoregulation. Also females have higher baseline heart rates at birth. These two factors may contribute to the observed differences in body temperature.

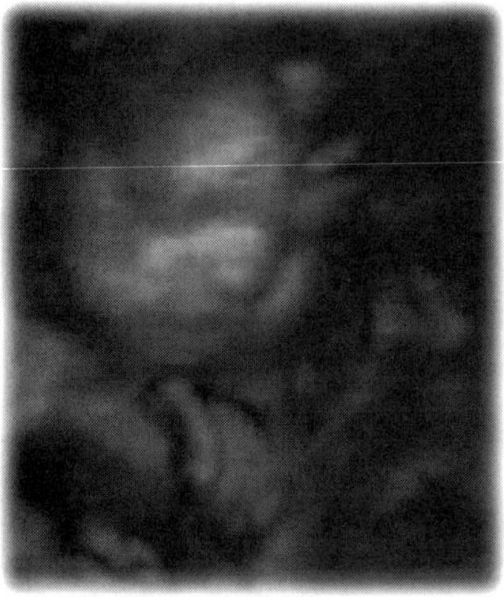

Thoughts:

....

....

DAY 251

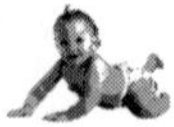

Do babies hear music the same way as adults? Studies measuring the brain activity of babies using functional magnetic resonance imaging (fMRI) showed that when music was played, measures of brain activation increased. In particular, the babies showed increased activity in the frontal and temporal lobes of the brain in the precise pattern that adults show listening to the same music. So based on the pattern of brain activation, it is suggested that babies do hear music as we do.

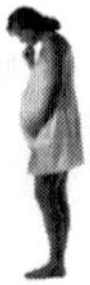

Lightening is the term used to refer to when the baby 'drops' into the pelvic girdle in preparation for birth. You'll notice that it's easier to breathe and your stomach won't feel as full after eating because the baby has shifted downward. The baby can drop anywhere from 2 - 4 weeks prior to birth.

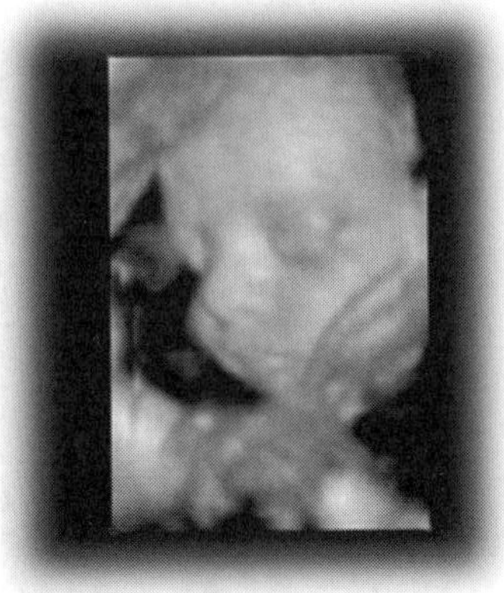

Notes:

....

....

The baby's brain responds more to light flashes when it's in dream sleep (REM) compared to quiet or non-REM sleep. Sensitive measurements of the retina's response to light showed a larger response when the baby is in REM sleep. One inference from this finding is that environmentally and internally generated visual signals - the visual component of dreams familiar to us - are components of your baby's dreams as well. Also, since the brain is growing during REM sleep, these visual signals may play a role in the development and maturation of the visual system.

Uterine contractions are forceful. Over 50 lbs of pressure is applied during each contraction. The force is spread out and the baby is buffered by the amniotic fluid. The forceful contractions are necessary to force open the cervix and push the baby out.

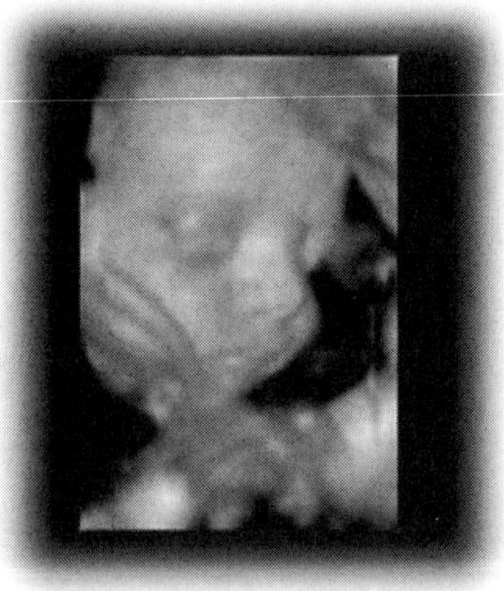

Thoughts:

....

....

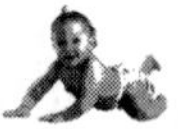

Sometimes the characteristics of one behavior can predict another. In this case scientists studied the movement patterns of fetuses at 37 weeks and found that aspects of the behavior was related to later crying behavior after birth. Strong movements (kicking, trunk movements, whole body shifts) did not predict later crying. However, weak movements defined as hand movements, arm movements and minor position shifts, which may be an indication of general activity level, did relate to crying at 1, 6 and 12 weeks after birth. Fetuses that showed more of these weak movements cried more. The mechanism of the difference is unknown but could be related to individual differences in overall reactivity levels to stimulation.

Baby is 22 inches ❦ 7.0 lbs.

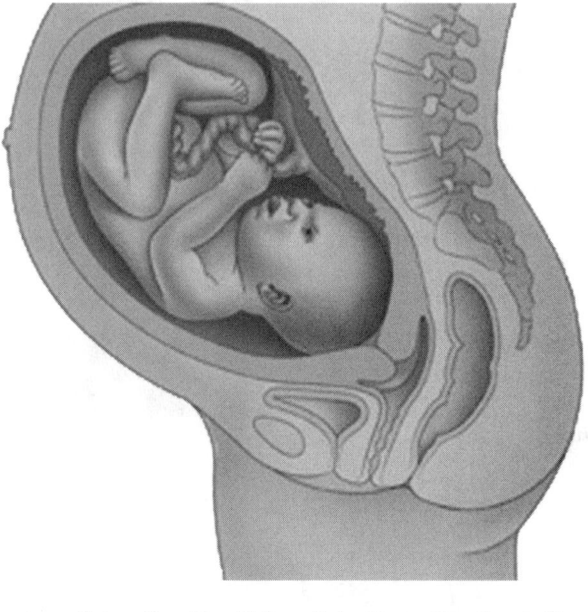

DAY 254

Amniotic fluid has substances in it that the baby can detect using its chemical senses (taste and olfaction/smell). An interesting study has shown that amniotic fluid odor can be detected by newborns and that it has a calming effect on them. Babies exposed to the odor of amniotic fluid cried significantly less when separated from mother compared to babies exposed to the mother's breast odor or no odor. Amniotic fluid odors may have a calming effect because it provides a degree of familiarity in the very novel extrauterine world. Just wait until your child needs her blankie or suckie (pacifier) to calm down and go to sleep.

Any day now you'll have a new baby, and if this is your first, you'll be a family.

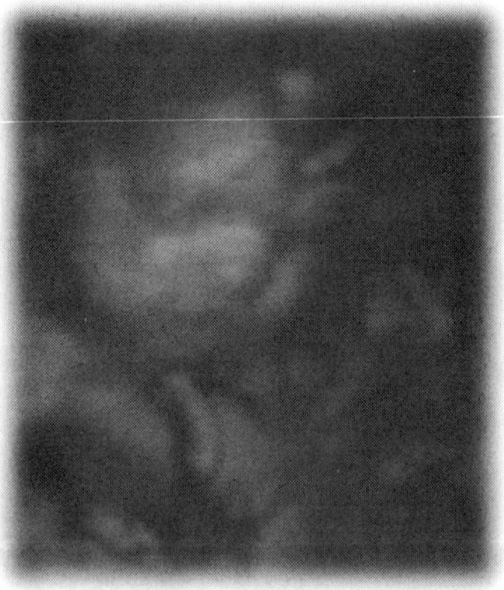

Thoughts:

....

....

DAY 255

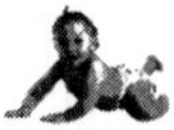

Babies have an inborn appreciation of how things should work in the world. In one study, babies observed two dolls being placed behind a screen. Then one group of babies observed another doll being placed behind the screen, while the other group was blocked from seeing the doll put behind the screen. The babies that observed the extra doll being placed behind the screen were not surprised to see 3 dolls when the screen was removed. The babies that only saw 2 dolls placed behind the screen were surprised to see 3 dolls when the screen was taken away, as shown by the length of time they studies the dolls. This study shows that the babies were keeping track of how many dolls were being placed behind the screen. Babies have an basic understanding of quantity.

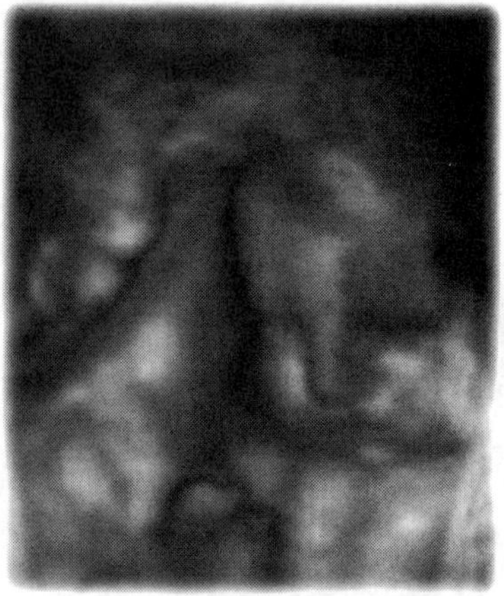

Notes:

....

....

DAY 256

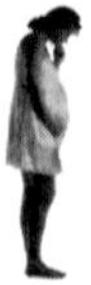

Without progesterone in your bloodstream, the uterine and abdominal muscles would contract to expel the fetus during pregnancy. Progesterone inhibits abdominal contractions and circulating estrogen is enough to keep muscles toned and ready to forcefully contract during labor. Over the last 3 weeks or so, your estrogen levels have increased, which has the effect of softening and effacing your cervix, enhancing muscle contractions and promoting blood clotting. Increased estrogen also leads to an increase in oxytocin receptors in your uterine and abdominal muscle. Oxytocin will cause the significantly different muscle contractions of labor. Oxytocin will be released from your brain's pituitary gland following a chemical signal from your baby that now is the time to be born.

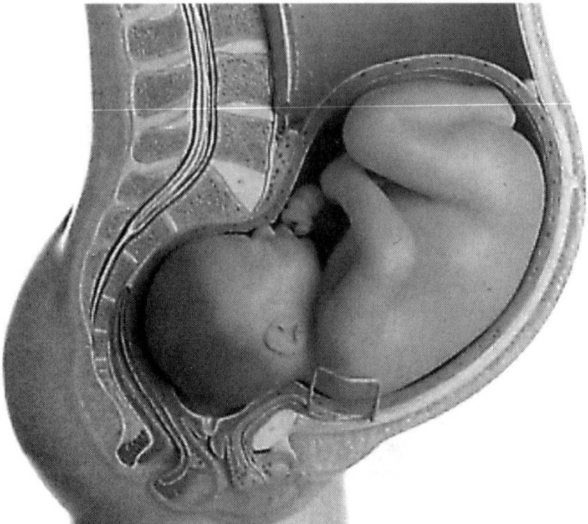

This is what the baby looks like with the head engaged in the cervix. You can see why your back might hurt a little.

DAY 257

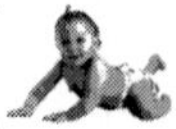

The laguno covering your baby's body has mostly come off and is suspended in the amniotic fluid. Your baby ingests the fluid along with the laguno hair. This has the effect of 'priming' the digestive tract in preparation for the processing of food. In fact, the stuff of the initial bowel movements of babies, also known as meconium, is made of laguno, colored green by bile from the gall bladder. The digestive tract is sterile now, however, bacteria which assist digestion, will be present in the intestines a few days after birth.

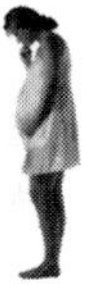

What to bring to the hospital: Bring a robe, ample nightgowns, warm socks, hair items (bands, brush), underwear, nursing bras, slippers, toiletries and any snacks you'll want that may not be available at the hospital. Also bring your baby name book (if you haven't yet decided), and going home outfits for you and the baby. And don't forget diapers, blankets and the car seat for the baby.

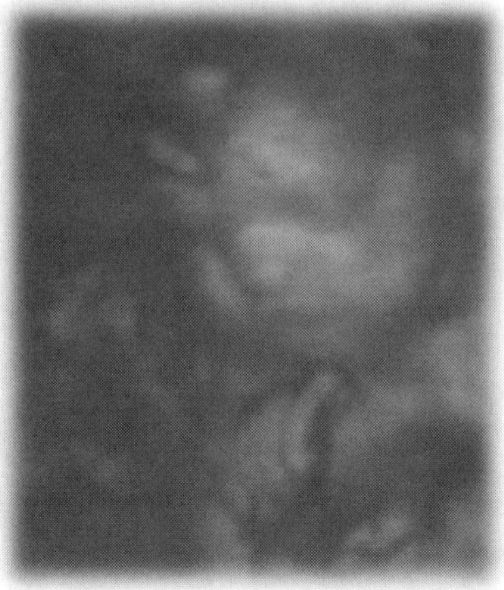

Notes:

....

....

DAY 258

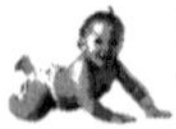

Uterine contractions in the form of Braxton-Hicks contractions produce increases in intrauterine pressure that 'squeeze' the baby. These contractions are detected by the baby because they typically show a slowing of heart rate during the contraction. Animal studies suggest that compression of the fetus, as occurs during these contractions and especially during the forceful expelling contractions of labor, are a key factor in initiating respiration upon birth.

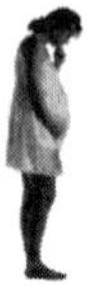

Your husband or support person should also prepare ahead of time for the big day. Be sure to keep enough gas in the car so you don't have to stop on the way to the hospital, and make sure that they can be reached easily by phone at all times. They'll also need some cash for the hospital cafeteria, parking garage and other small items while at the hospital.

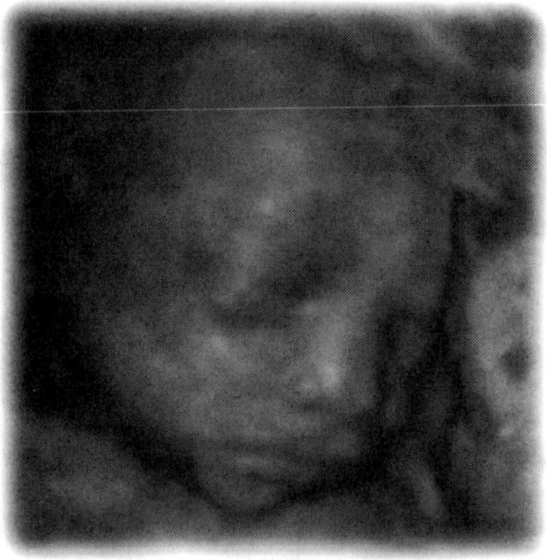

Thoughts:

....

....

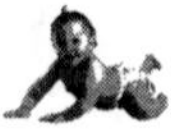

Breathing movements decrease up to the day of birth. Hiccups, even though they are very abrupt movements, don't cause state transitions in the baby. In other words, the baby won't wake up or shift from REM sleep to quiet sleep if they experience a bout of hiccups. Breathing behavior is also taking on a circadian rhythmicity. Breathing movements occur more often in the daylight hours (8am - 4pm) whereas hiccups occur in the nighttime hours (4pm - 8am).

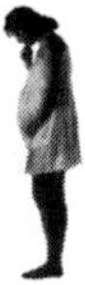

Epidural anesthesia involves direct administration of pain-blocking drugs to the spinal cord, stopping the transmission of the pain signals of labor and delivery to the brain. Studies have shown that women given epidurals are just as likely to deliver vaginally, so epidurals do not increase the likelihood of Caesarian section births.

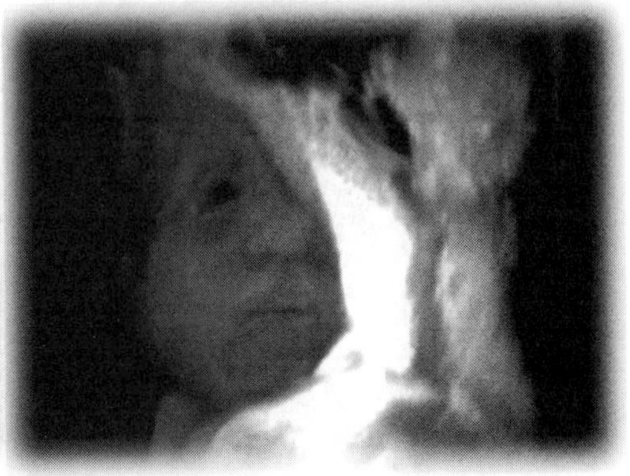

Notes:

....

....

DAY 260

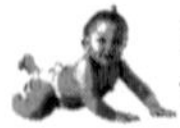

Babies show evidence of handedness as early as 12 weeks when they preferentially suck one thumb or the other (90% of the time it's the right thumb). Babies will also show a preference to lie with their heads turned to the right. Anatomical studies have found that the neural circuit that descends from the brain to the spinal cord is larger on one side vs. the other. In a right-handed person this simple anatomical difference would send more neural control to the right side of the body, particularly the arm and hand, making tasks 'easier' and more forceful by recruiting more motor neurons and muscle fibers with that hand.

Baby is 22 inches ❦ 7.5 lbs.

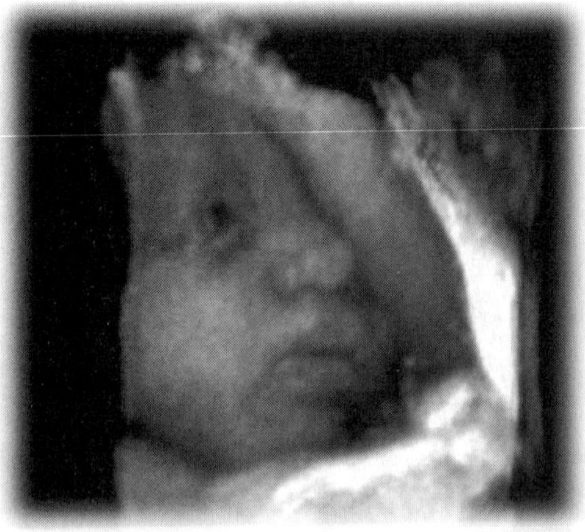

Thoughts:

DAY 261

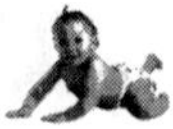

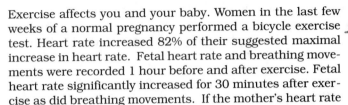

Exercise affects you and your baby. Women in the last few weeks of a normal pregnancy performed a bicycle exercise test. Heart rate increased 82% of their suggested maximal increase in heart rate. Fetal heart rate and breathing movements were recorded 1 hour before and after exercise. Fetal heart rate significantly increased for 30 minutes after exercise as did breathing movements. If the mother's heart rate increased in the 90%⁺ range, the baby's breathing movements decreased as did body movements. Heavy exercise affects the baby with signs of temporary fetal impairment

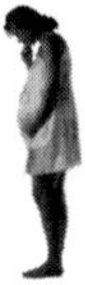

For unknown reasons, many women experience a burst of energy just before they go into labor. They will become very ambitious, perhaps cleaning, reorganizing etc. Save your energy...you'll need it for the birth and for your new baby.

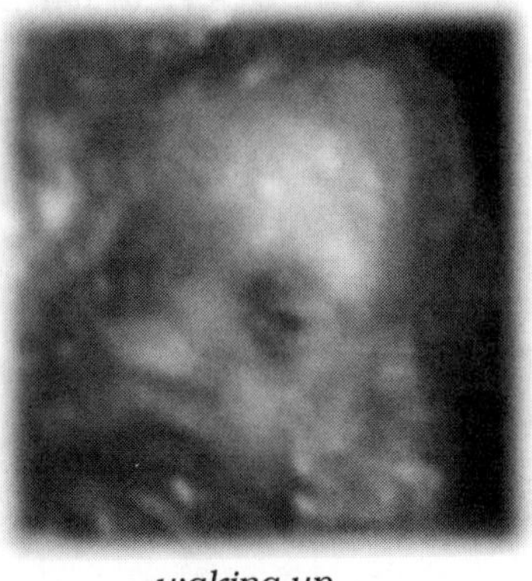

waking up

Notes:

....

....

DAY 262

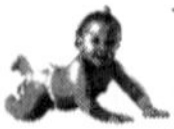

Your baby is adding about 14 grams (1/2 oz) of fat each day since about 35 weeks. The baby's body is about 16% body fat. The skin is normally a bluish-pink; and the testes in boys have descended into the scrotum.

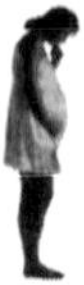

After birth, the stump of the umbilical cord will be swabbed with antibiotic and sometimes a plastic clothes pin-type clamp is attached after it is cut. The stump dries and shrivels up in about a week, and will fall off about 2 weeks later.

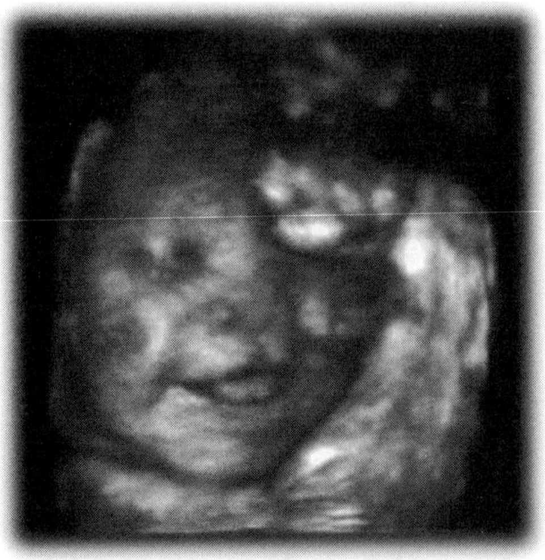

Thoughts:

....

....

DAY 263

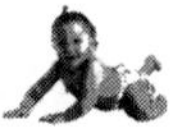

Your baby's brain will weigh about 14 oz at birth. By the time your baby is 1 year old her brain will weigh 20 ounces, and by 6 years it will be 45 ounces. Clearly the brain is increasing in size and weight. All of this extra neural apparatus serves an adaptive function, otherwise it wouldn't be there. One reason why the brain continues to grow postnatally is that a 45 oz or even a 20 oz brain would be almost impossible to squeeze through your pelvis. So the solution nature has derived is to extend the brain development period outside the womb. Some scientists think the human gestation period is closer to 21 months rather than 9. According to this theory, infants are externalized fetuses with truly amazing capabilities.

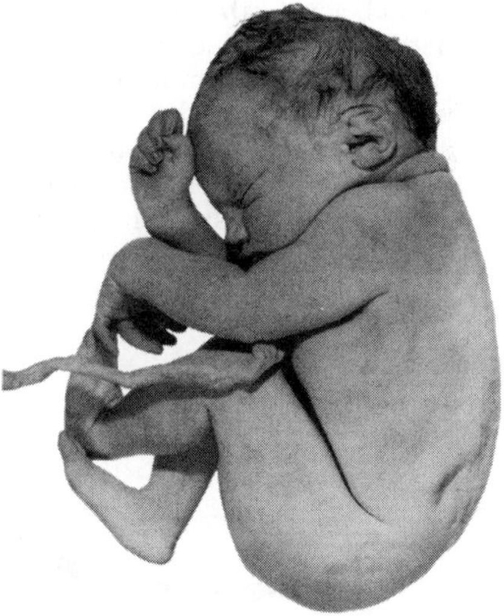

Notes:

....

....

DAY 264

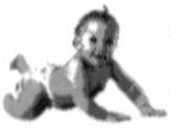

85% of babies are born within two weeks of their projected due date. So it could happen any day now.

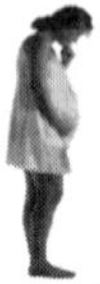

Your cervix will eventually dilate or open to 10 centimeters right before birth. As a reference, the circle shown here is 10 centimeters in diameter. The cervix dilates due to the thinning and shortening of the cervical canal during the course of labor. The birth canal is composed of a bony pelvis and the soft tissues of the cervix and vagina. The canal is not smooth and straight but resembles a curved tube with ridges.

Thoughts:

....

....

DAY 265

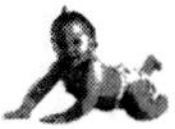

Studies have shown that women who expressed more affection towards their unborn baby displayed more confidence in their new role and showed better postpartum adjustment with their baby. Mothers in the last trimester of pregnancy were asked questions from the Prenatal Attachment Inventory PAI (which describes the mother's thoughts, feelings & relationship to the fetus). Later the mother's interactions with the baby were assessed by direct observation of the mother and infant 12 weeks after birth. Mothers who scored higher on the PAI (showed greater affection and fantasized more about the baby) showed more involvement with their babies at 12 weeks. These mothers were more active - stimulating their babies more and engaging in more face-to-face interaction. And the babies of these mothers were more responsive and interactive (smiling, vocalizing, looking at mother) as well.

Prenatal Attachment Inventory

Factors	Sample items
Fantasy	I wonder what my baby looks like now I dream about the baby
Interaction	I know when my baby is asleep I can make my baby move
Affection	I feel love for the baby I enjoy feeling the baby move
Baby as distinct from self	I think my baby already has a personality I imagine calling baby by name
Sharing pleasures	I tell others what the baby is doing I let others put their hands on my belly

from Mueller (1993).

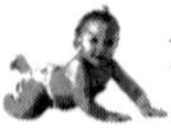

Any day now your baby will be born. Remember that your baby will choose its birthdate by initiating the mechanisms of labor.

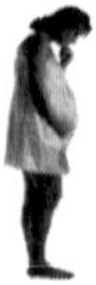

Also remember that your due date was estimated assuming that you had a 28-day menstrual cycle. If your cycle is shorter or longer than 28 days you're due date could vary accordingly. Most health care practitioner's today won't allow your pregnancy to go two weeks beyond your due date. If these two weeks pass your practitioner may take measures to help induce labor. At the hospital they may apply a gel rich in prostaglandins to your cervix to soften it. You could also receive Pitocin intravenously to stimulate uterine contractions.

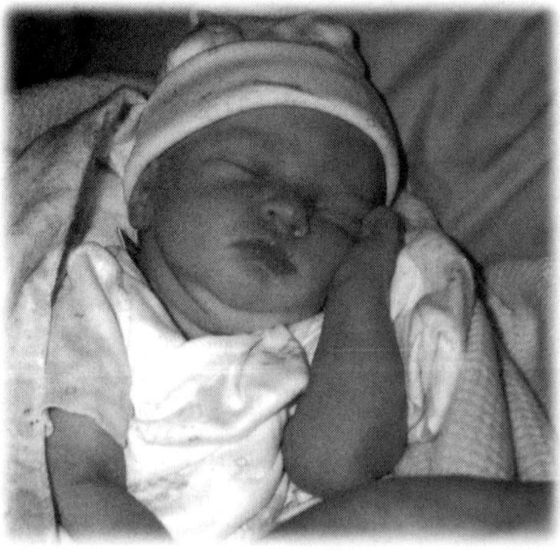

One goal of this book, in addition to providing lots of useful information on your baby's progress, was to help foster the relationship between you and your baby. We tried to do this by simply making the unseen seen. Motherhood is the continuation of an already existing affectionate relationship between you and your baby. Many studies have shown that mothers experience a growing affection and attachment to their developing baby during pregnancy. Most women report a mental image of what their unborn baby looks like at around 3 months gestation. Then after the first quickening movements are felt, there is a rapid increase in measured attachment. When a definite pattern of rest and activity is recognized, mothers respond to their baby in an increasingly synchronized fashion. All of this translates into increased feelings of affection for the baby.

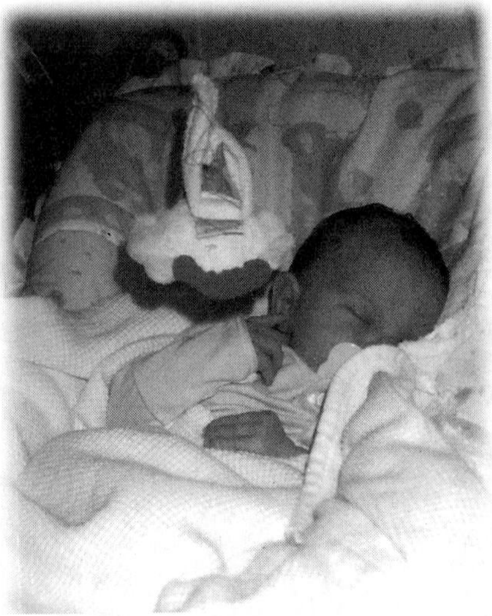

Enjoy your new baby!

Further Reading

This section explains some of the finer attributes of the behavioral procedures used to assess the competencies of the unborn and newborn baby throughout this book.

Habituation: The decrement in attention directed toward a source of stimulation. With babies or fetuses outside the womb, an experimenter would place the child in a seat as in the photo, and measure various responses. These responses can be visual fixation (how long the baby looks at it), autonomic responses like heart rate, blood pressure or other responses, or neural responses like evoked brain potentials. When the image first appears, the baby orients to the screen and she looks at it. If the same image is presented over and over the baby's attention directed to it will decrease. They will look at the image less and less. The measurement of this decrease in looking over repeated presentations of a stimulus is called habituation.

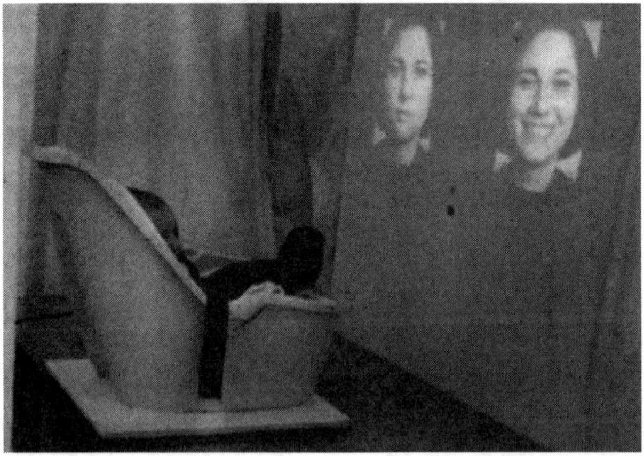

from Bornstein (1998).

There is a wealth of information gained from this simple testing procedure. Scientists can measure perceptual discrimination behavior (seeing the difference between things), attention, short-term memory, long-term memory, and the capacity of the child to learn. All without requiring the child to say a single word; their visual, and autonomic behavior indicates to the scientist what the baby knows.

Non-nutritive sucking: Babies are proficient at sucking. The procedure involves fitting the baby with earphones and a nipple that measures the rate of sucking. When babies hear certain sounds they express their preferences by changing their vigor and rhythm of sucking. Babies increase their sucking when they prefer what they are hearing. This is the test that demonstrated babies prefer their mother's voice. The test is a way to measure preferences using the voluntary sucking behavior, and it is used to test memory and learning.

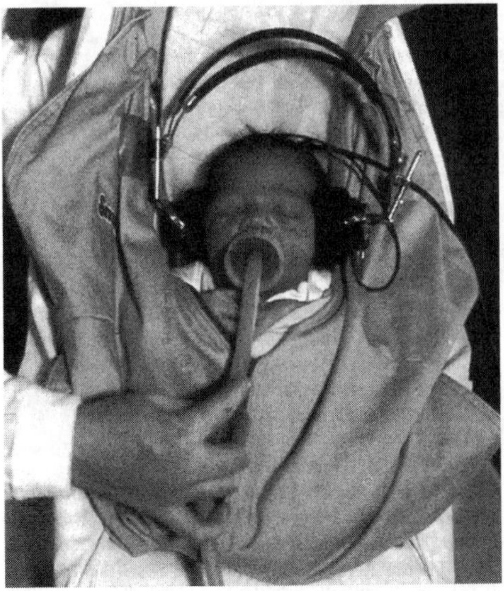

from Fifer and Moon (1989).

Autonomic orienting responses: The heart is under neural control from the brain. Sensory stimuli (sounds, visual images, smells, tastes, touches) are relayed to the brain and the brain influences the heart through the vagus nerve, among other nerves. Recording the activity of the heart is an easy behavioral measure of the response of the brain to a variety of environmental stimuli. Usually in response to a sound the heart rate slows down due to increased activity in the vagus nerve. This heart slowing response is considered a component of an orienting, or "what-is-it" response. Responses like the heart rate response provide scientists a way to ask if a non-verbal baby can detect and attend to stimuli in their environment.

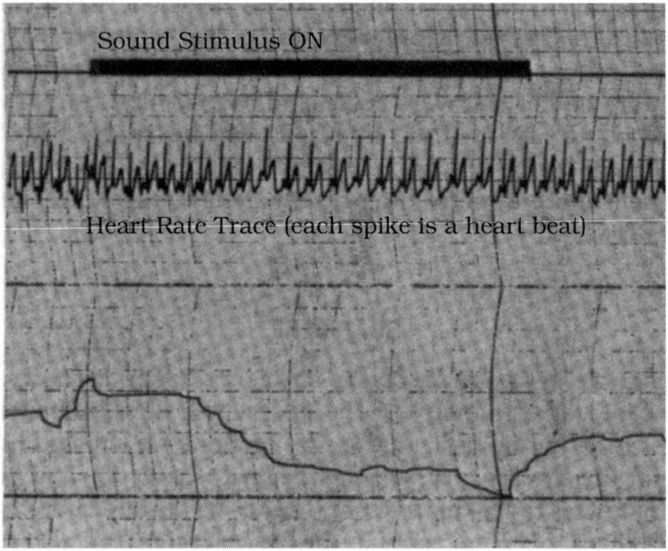

Measurement of the interval between each beat (as the trace goes down the time between the beats is lengthening which means the heart is slowing). In this example, a sound is played and the heart rate slows down. This is evidence that the baby heard the sound and attended to it. Scientists can also use heart rate measurements to study learning and memory.

Ultrasound Recordings: Ultrasounds are images created by the reflection of sound waves off a solid object back to the transducer or recorder. The readings are fed into a computer that can perform very fast averaging of the information and produce real-time images of what the baby looks like and is doing. Most women in the United States will have an ultrasound exam between the 16th and 20th weeks of pregnancy. The procedure will be used to pinpoint the date of the pregnancy based on the baby's size, locate the placement of the placenta, measure the amount of amniotic fluid and assess the general well-being of the baby.

Newer 3-D ultrasounds show the baby in greater detail. Presenting a realistic image with depth and substance. Even newer 4-D ultrasounds shows how your baby moves and the images are presented in real-time...as they are happening!

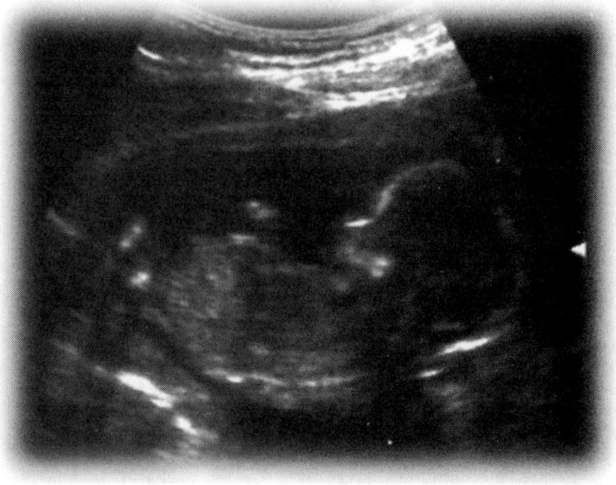

References

Alley, T.R. (1981). Head shape and the perception of cuteness. Developmental Psychology, 17, 650-654.

Als, H. (1985). Patterns of infant behavior: Analogues of later organizational difficulties? In F. H. Duffy & N. Geschwind (Eds.), Dyslexia: A neuroscientific approach to clinical evaluation (pp. 67-92). Boston: Little, Brown.

Als, H., & Duffy, F. H. (1983). The behavior of the premature infant: A theoretical framework for a systematic assessment. In T. B. Brazelton & B. M. Lester (Eds.), New approaches to developmental screening of infants (pp. 153-174). New York: Elsevier, North Holland.

Als, H., Duffy, F. H., & McAnulty, G. B. (1988a). Behavioral differences between preterm and fullterm newborns as measured with the A.P.I.B. system scores: I. Infant Behavior and Development, 11, 305-318.

Als, H., Duffy, F. H., & McAnulty, G. B. (1988b). The A.P.I.B.: An assessment of functional competence in preterm and fullterm newborns regardless of gestational age at birth: II. Infant Behavior and Development, 11, 319-331.

Als, H., Duffy, F. H., McAnulty, G., & Badian, N. (1989). Continuity of neurobehavioral functioning in preterm and full-term newborns. In M. H. Bornstein & N. A. Krasnegor (Eds.), Stability and continuity in mental development (pp.3-28). Hillsdale, NJ: Lawrence Erlbaum Associates.

Amir, L. H. (2001). Maternal smoking and reduced duration of breastfeeding: a review of possible mechanisms. Early Human Development, 65, 45-67.

Bang, B. G. (1964). The mucous glands of the developing human nose. Acta Anatomica, 59, 297-314.

Barcroft, J., & Mason, M. F. (1938). The atmosphere in which the foetus lives. Journal of Physiology (London), 93, P22.

Bertenthal, B., Campos, J & Haith, M. (1980). Development of visual organization: Perception of subjective contours. Child Development, 51, 1072-1080.

Birnholz, J. C., & Benacerraf, B. R. (1983). The development of human fetal hearing Science, 222, 516-518.

Blakemore, C., & Cooper, G. F. (1970). Development of brain depends on the visual environment. Nature, 228, 477-478.

Boklage, C. E. (1980). The sinistral blastocyst: An embryonic perspective on the development of brain function asymmetries. In J. Herron (Ed.), Neuropsychology of left-handedness (pp. 115-137). NY: Academic Press.

Bossy J. (1980). Development of olfactory and related structures in staged human embryos. Anatomy and Embryology, 161, 225-236.

Bornstein, M.H. & Tamis-LeMonda, C.S. (1990). Activities and interaction of mothers and their firstborn infants in the first six months of life: covariation, stability, continuity, correspondence, and prediction. Child Development, 61, 1206-1217.

Bornstein, M.H. (1998) Stability in mental development from early life:methods, measures, meanings and myths. In Simion, F and Butterworth, G. (Eds.), The Development of Sensory, Motor and Cognitive Capacities in Early Infancy: From Perception to Cognition, Psychology Press, 301-333.

Bradley R. M., & Mistretta C. M. (1971). Intravascular taste in rats as demonstrated by conditioned aversion to sodium saccharin. Journal of Comparative and Physiological Psychology, 75,186-189.

Bradley, R. M., & Mistretta, C. M. (1975). Fetal sensory receptors. Physiological Reviews, 55, 352-382

Brookover, C. (1914). The peripheral distribution of the nervus terminalis in an infant. Journal of Comparative Neurology, 28, 349-360.

Brown, J. W. (1974). Prenatal development of the human chief sensory trigeminal nucleus. Journal of Comparative Neurology, 156, 307-336.

Brunjes P. C., & Frazier, L. L. (1986). Maturation and plasticity in the olfactory system of vertebrates. Brain Research Reviews, 11,1-45.

Bryden, M. P., & Steenhuis, R. E. (1991). Issues in the assessment of handedness. In F. L. Kitterle (Ed.), Cerebral laterality (pp.35-51). Hillsdale, NJ: Lawrence Erlbaum Associates.

Burroughs, A. K., Asonye, U. O., Anderson-Shanklin, G. C., & Vidyasagar, D. (1978). The effect of non-nutritive sucking on transcutaneous oxygen tension in non-crying preterm neonates. Research in Nursing and Health, 1, 69-75.

Carmichael, L. (1970). Onset and early development of behavior. In P. H. Mussen (Ed.), Manual of child psychology (Vol. 1., pp. 447-563). New York: Wiley.

Case, R. (1992). The role of the frontal lobes in the regulation of cognitive development. Brain and Cognition, 20, 51-73.

Cauna, N., Hinderer, K. & Wentges, R. T. (1969). Sensory receptor organs of the human respiratory mucosa. American Journal of Anatomy, 124, 607-612.

Caza, P.A., & Spear, N. E. (1984). Short-term exposure to an odor increases its subsequent preference in preweanling rats: A descriptive profile of the phenomenon. Developmental Psychobiology, 17, 407-422.

Chaudhari, S., Kulkarni, S., Pajnigar, F., Pandit, A. N., & Deshmukh, S. (1991). A longitudinal follow up of development of preterm infants. Indian Pediatrics, 28, 873-880.

Chi, J. G., Dooling, E. C., & Gilles, F. H. (1977). Gyral development of the human brain. Journal of Neurology, 1, 86-93.

Chi,J. G.,Dooling, E. C., & Gilles,F. H. (1977). Left-right asymmetries of the temporal speech area of the human fetus. Arch of Neurology, 34, 346-348.

Clarkson, M. G., & Berg, W. K. (1983). Cardiac orienting and vowel discrimination in newborns: Crucial stimulus parameters. Child Development, 54,162-171.

Condon, W. S. & Sander, L. W. (1974) Neonate movement is synchronized to adult speech: interactional participation and language acquisition. Science, 183, 99-101.

Coppola, D. M., & O'Connell, R. J. (1989). Stimulus access to olfactory and vomeronasal receptors in utero. Neuroscience Letters, 106, 241-248.

Crook, C. (1987). Taste and olfaction. In P. Salapatek & L. Cohen, L. (Eds.), Handbook of infant perception: Vol. 1. From sensation to perception (pp.237-264). Orlando, FL: Academic Press.

Cowan, W. M. (1979). The development of the brain. Scientific Am, 241, 113-131.

Cupoli, J. M., Gagan, R. J., Watkins, A. H., & Bell, S. F. (1986). The shapes of grief. Journal of Perinatology, 6, 123-126.

Dancis, J. (1978). The placenta: An overview. In U. Stawe (Ed.), Perinatal physiology (pp. 19-26). New York: Plenum.

Davidson, R. J. (1992). Anterior cerebral asymmetry and the nature of emotion. Brain and Cognition, 20,125-151.

Davidson, R. J., & Fox, N. A. (1989). Frontal brain assymmetry predicts infants' response to maternal separation. Journal of Abnormal Psychology, 98,127-131.

Dawson, G., Panagioddes, H., Klinger, L. G., & Hill, D. (1992). The role of frontal lobe functioning in the development of infant self-regulatory behavior. Brain and Cognition, 20, 152-175.

DeCasper, A. J., & Carstens, A. A. (1981). Contingencies of stimulation:Effects on learning and emotion in neonates. Infant Bev & Dev, 4,19-35.

DeCasper, A. J., & Fifer, W. P. (1980). Of human bonding: Newborns prefer their mothers' voices. Science, 208,1174 1176.

DeCasper, A. J., & Sigafoos, A. D. (1983). The intrauterine heartbeat: A potent reinforcer for newborns. Infant Behavior and Development, 6,19-25.
DeCasper, A. J., & Spence, M. J. (1986). Prenatal maternal speech influences newborns'perception of speech sounds. Infant Behavior and Development, 9,133-150.
DeCasper, A. J., & Spence, M. J. (1991). Auditorily mediated behavior during the perinatal period: A cognitive view. In M. J. Weiss & P. R. Zelazo(Eds.), Newborn attention: Biological constraints and the influence of experience.
D'Elia, A., Pighetti, M., Moccia, G. & Santangelo, N. (2001). Spontaneous motor activity in normal fetuses. Early Human Development, 65, 139-147.
Devoe, L. D., Murray, C., Faircloth, D., & Ramos, E. (1990). Vibroacoustic stimulation and fetal behavioural state in normal term human pregnancy. AmericanJournal of Obstetrics and Gynecology, 163, 1156-1161.
DeVries, J. I. P., Visser, G. H. A., & Prechtl, H. F. R. (1982). The emergence of fetal behaviour: 1. Qualitative aspects. Early Human Development, 7, 301-322.
Divon, M. Y., Platt, L. D., Cantrell, C. J., Smith, C. V., Yeh, S. Y. Y., & Paul, R. H. (1985). Evoked fetal startle response: A possible intrauterine neurological examination. American Journal of Obstetrics and Gynecology, 153, 454-456.
DiPietro, J.A. et al. (1996). Development of fetal movement: fetal heart-rate coupling from 20 wks through term. Early Human Dev., 44, 139-151.
Dooling, E. C., Chi, J. G., & Gilles, F. H. (1983). Telencephalic development: Changing gyral patterns. In F. H. Gilles, A. Leviton, & E. C. Dooling (Eds.), The developing human brain: Growth and epidemiologic neuropathy (pp. 94-104). Boston: J. Wright.
Doty, R. L. (1992). Olfactory function in neonates. In D. G. Laing, R. L. Doty, & W. Breipohl (Eds.), The human sense of smell (pp. 155-165). Berlin: Springer Verlag.
Dreyfus-Brisac, C. (1975). Neurophysiological studies in human premature and full-term infants. Biological Psychiatry, 10, 485-495.
Dreyfus-Brisac, C., Fischgold, H., Samson-Dollfus, D., Sainte-Anne Dargassies, S., Monod, N., & Blanc, C. (1957). Veille, sommeil, reactivite sensorielle chez le premature, le nouveau-ne et le nourrison. Electroencephalography and Clinical Neurophysiology, 6, (Suppl.), 418-440.
Duclaux, R., Challamel, M. J., Collet, L., Roullet-Solignac, I., & Revoli, M. (1991). Hemispheric asymmetry of late auditory evoked response induced by pitch changes in infants: Influence of sleep stages. Brain Research, 566,152-158
Duenholter, J. H., & Pritchard, J. A. (1976). Fetal respiration: Quantitative measurements of amniotic fluid inspired near term by human and rhesus fetuses. American Journal of Obstetrics and Gynecology, 125, 306-309.
Duffy, F. H., Als, H., & McAnulty, G. B. (1990). Behavioral and electrophysiological evidence for gestational age effects in healthy preterm and fullterm infants studied two weeks after expected due date. Child Development, 61,1271-1286.
Duffy, F. H., Burchfiel, J. L., & Lombroso, C. T. (1979). Brain electrical activity mapping (BEAM): A method for extending the clinical ablity of EEG and evoked potential data. Annals of Neurology, 5, 309-321.
Duffy, F. H., Mower, G. D., Jensen, F., & Als, H. (1984). Neural plasticity: A new frontier for infant development. In H. E. Fitzgerald, B. M. Lester, & M. W. Yogman (Eds.), Theory and research in behavioral pediatrics (pp.67-96). New York: Plenum.
Engel, R., & Benson, R. C. (1968). Estimate of conceptional age by evoked response activity. Biologia Neonatorum, 12, 201-213.
Farbman, A. I. (1986). Prenatal development of mammalian olfactory receptor cells. Chemical Senses, 11, 3-18.

Fantz, R. L. (1963). Pattern vision in newborn infants. Science, 140, 296-297
Ferrari, F., Grosoli, M. V., Fontana, G., & Cavazzuti, G. B. (1983). Neurobehavioral comparison of low-risk preterm and fullterm infants at term conceptual age. Dev Medicine & Child Neurology, 25, 450 458.
Field, T. M., Ignatoff, E., Stringer, S., Brennan, J., Greenberg, R., & Anderson, G. (1982). Non-nutritive sucking during tube feedings: Effects on preterm neonates in an intensive care unit. Pediatrics, 70(3), 381-384.
Fifer, W. P., & Moon, C. (1989). Psychobiology of newborn auditory preferences. Seminars in Perinatology, 13(5), 430-433.
Finlay, B. L., & Miller, B. (1993). Regressive events in early cortical maturation: Their significance for the outcome of early brain damage. In A. M. Galaburda (Ed.), Dyslexia & Development. Cambridge, MA: Harvard University Press.
Fischer, K. W., & Rose, S. T. (1994). Dynamic development of coordination of components in brain and behavior: A framework for theory and research. In G. Dawson & K. W. Fischer (Eds.), Human behavior and the developing brain (pp.3 66). New York: Guilford.
Flanagan, Geraldine L. (1962). The First Nine Months of Life. New York: Simon & Schuster.
Fox, R. & McDaniel, C. (1982). The perception of biological motion by human infants. Science, 218, 486-487.
Fox, N. A. (1991). If it's not left, it's right. American Psychologist, 46, 863-872.
Fox, N. A., & Bell, M. (1990). Electrophysiological indices of frontal lobe development: Relations for cognitive and affective behavior in human infants over the first year of life. Annals of the NY Acad of Sciences, 608, 677-698.
Fuller, J. R. (1989). Early patterns of maternal attachment. Health Care for Women Int., 11, 433-446.
Gagnon, R. (1989). Stimulation of human fetuses with sound and vibration. Seminars in Perinatology, 13, 393-402.
Gagnon, R., Benzaquen, S., & Hunse, C. (1992). The fetal sound environment during vibroacoustic stimulation in labour, Effect on fetal heart rate response. Obstetrics and Gynecology, 79, 905-955.
Gagnon, R., Foreman, J., Hunse, C., & Patrick, J. (1989). Effects of low-frequency vibration on human term fetus. American Journal of Obstetrics and Gynecology, 161,1479-1476.
Gagnon, R., Hunse, C., & Bocking, A. D. (1989b). Fetal heart rate patterns in the small-for-gestational-age human fetus. American Journal of Obstetrics and Gynecology, 161, 779-784.
Gagnon, R., Hunse, C., Carmichael, L., Fellows, F., & Patrick, J. (1987). Human fetal response to vibratory acoustic stimulation from twenty-six weeks to term. American Journal of Obstetrics and Gynecology, 157,1375-1381.
Gagnon, R., Hunse, C., Carmichael, L., Fellows, F., & Patrick, J. (1988). Fetal heart rate and fetal activity patterns after vibratory acoustic stimulation at thirty to thirty-two weeks' gestational age. American Journal of Obstetrics and Gynecology, 158, 75-79.
Gagnon, R., Hunse, C., Carmichael, L., & Patrick, J. (1989). Vibratory acoustic stimulation in 26- to 32-week, small-for-gestational-age fetus. American Journal of Obstetrics and Gynecology, 160,160-165.
Gagnon, R., Patrick, J., Foreman, J., & West, R. (1986). Stimulation of human fetuses with sound and vibration. American Journal of Obstetrics and Gynecology, 155, 848-851.
Gagnon, R., Hunse, C., & Patrick, J. (1988). Fetal responses to vibratory acoustic stimulation, Influence of basal heart rate. American Journal of Obstetrics and Gynecology, 159, 835-839.
Geschwind, N., & Galaburda, A. S. (1987). Cerebral lateralization. Cambridge, MA: MIT Press.

Geschwind, N., & Levitsky, W. (1968). Human brain: Left right asymmetries in temporal speech region. Science, 161,186-187.
Gilles, F. H., Leviton, A., & Dooling, E. C. (1983). The developing human brain. Boston: John Wright.
Goodwin, R. S., & Michel, G. F. (1981). Head orientation position during birth and in infant neonatal period, and hand preference at nineteen weeks. Child Development, 52, 819-826.
Gorski, P. A., Hole, W. T., Leonard, C. H., & Martin, J. A. (1983). Direct computer recording of premature infants and nursery care: Distress following two interventions. Pediatrics, 72, 198-202.
Gottlieb, G. (1971). Ontogenesis of sensory function in birds and mammals. In E. Tobach, L. R. Aronson, & E. Shaw (Eds.), The biopsychology of development (pp.67-128). New York: Academic Press.
Graham, F. K., Anthony, B. J., & Zeigler, B. L. (1983). The orienting response and developmental processes. In D. Siddle (Ed.), Orienting and habituation: Perspectives in human research (pp. 371-430). UK: Wiley, Sussex.
Granier-Deferre, C., Lecanuet, J. P., Cohen, H., & Busnel, M. C. (1983). Preliminary evidence on fetal auditory habituation. In G. Rossi (Ed.), Noise as a public health problem (Vol. 1, pp. 561-572). Milan, Italy: Edizioni.
Greenough, W. T. (1975). Experimental modification of the developing brain. American Scientist, 63, 37-46.
Greenough, W. T. (1986). What's special about development? Thoughts on the bases of experience-sensitive synaptic plasticity. In W. T. Greenough & J. M. Juraska (Eds.), Developmental neuropsychology. New York:Academic Press.
Grimwade, J. C., Walker, D. W., Bartlett, M., Gordon, S., & Wood, C. (1971). Human fetal heart rate change and movement in response to sound and vibration. American Journal of Obstetrics and Gynecology, 109, 86-90.
Groome, L.J et al. (1999). Behavioral state affects heart rate response to low-intensity sound in human fetuses. Early Human Development, 54, 39-54.
Gluckman, P. D., Gunn, T. R., & Johnston, B. M. (1983). The effects of cooling on breathing and shivering in unanesthaetized fetal lamb in utero. Journal of Physiology (London), 343, 495-506.
Hamburger, V. (1963). Some aspects of the embryology of behavior. Quarterly Review of Biology, 38, 342-365.
Harris, L. J. (1983). Laterality of function in the infant: Historical and contemporary trends in theory and research. In G. Young, S. J. Segalowitz, C. M. Corter, & S. E. Trehub (Eds.), Manual specialisation and the developing brain (pp. 177-247). New York: Academic Press.
Harris, L. J., & Carlson, D. F. (1988). Pathological left-handedness: An analysis of theories and evidence. In D. F. Molfese & S. J. Segalowitz (Eds.), Brain lateralization in children (pp. 289-372). New York: Guilford.
Henschall, W. R. (1972). Intrauterine sound levels. Journal of Obstetrics and Gynecology, 112, 577-579.
Hepper, P. G. (1987). The amniotic fluid: An important priming role in kin recognition. Animal Behavior, 35,1343-1346.
Hepper, P. G. (1988). Adaptive fetal learning: Prenatal exposure to garlic affects postnatal preferences. Animal Behavior, 36, 935-936.
Hepper, P. G. (1990). Fetal behaviour. A potential diagnostic tool. Midwifery, 6,193-200.
Hepper, P. G., & Shahidullah, S. (1992). Habituation in normal and Down syndrome fetuses. Quarterly Journal of Exp. Psychology, 44B, 305-317.
Hepper, P. G., Shahidullah, S., & White, R. (1991). Handedness in the human fetus. Neuropsychologia, 29,1107-1111.
Herlenius, E & Langercrantz, H. (2001). Neurotransmitters and neuromodulators during development. Early Human Development, 65, 21-37.

Hofer, M. A. (1981). The roots of human behavior: An introduction to the psychobiology of early human development. San Francisco: W. H. Freeman.

Hogg, I.D. (1941). Sensory nerves and associated structures in the skin of human fetuses of 8 to 14 weeks of menstrual age correlated with functional capacity. Journal of Comparative Neurology, 75, 371-410

Hooker, D. (1952) *The prenatal origin of behavior.* 18th Porter Lecture Series. Lawrence KS: Univ of Kansas Press.

Humphrey, T. (1964) Some correlations between the appearance of human fetal reflexes and the development of the nervous system. Progress in Brain Research, 4, 93-133.

Jensen, O. H. (1984). Fetal heart rate response to controlled sound stimuli during the third trimester of normal pregnancy. Acta Obstetrics et Gynecologica Scandinavica, 63, 193-197.

Jeffrey, W. E., & Cohen, L. B. (1971). Habituation in the human infant. Advances in Child Development, 3, 3-45.

Johnson, M.H. (1990). Cortical maturation and the development of visual attention in early infancy. Journal of Cognitive Neuroscience, 2, 81-95.

Johnson, M.H., Dziurawiec, S., Ellis, H., & Morton, J. (1991). Newborns' preferential tracking of face-like stimuli and its subsequent decline. Cognition, 40, 1-19.

Kenny, P. A., & Turkewitz, G. (1986). Effects of unusually early visual stimulation on the development of homing behavior in the rat pup. Developmental Psychobiology, 19, 57-66.

Kestenbaum, R & Nelson, C.A. (1990). The recognition and categorization of upright and inverted emotional expressions by 7-month-old infants. Infant Behavior and Development, 13, 497-511.

Kitterle, F. L. (Ed.). (1991). Cerebral laterality. Hillsdale, NJ: Lawrence Erlbaum Associates.

Kleiner, K.A. (1987). Amplitude and phase spectra as indices of infants' pattern preferences. Infant Behavior and Development, 10, 49-59.

Kuo, Z. Y. (1932). Ontogeny of embryonic behavior in Aves: I. The chronology and general nature of the behavior of the chick embryo. Journal of Experimental Zoology, 61, 395-430.

Kurtzberg, D., Hilpert, P. L., Kreuzer, J. A., & Vaughan, H. G., Jr. (1984). Differential maturation of cortical auditory evoked potentials to speech sounds in normal fullterm and very low-birthweight infants. Developmental Medicine and Child Neurology, 26, 466 475.

Kurtzberg, D., Stapells, D. R., & Wallace, I. F. (1988). Event related potential assessment of auditory system integrity: Implications for language development. In P. M. Vietz & H. G. Vaughan (Eds.), Early identification of infants with developmental disability (pp. 160-180). Philadelphia: Grune and Stratton.

Leader, L. R., Baille, P., Martin, B., & Vermeulen, E. (1982). The assessment and significance of habituation to a repeated shmulus by the human foetus. Early Human Development, 7, 211-219.

Leader, L. R., Baille, P., Martin, B., & Vermeulen, E. (1982). Foetal habituation in high risk pregnancies. British Journal of Obstetrics and Gynaecology, 89, 441-446.

Leader, L. R., Baillie, P., Martin, B., & Vermeulen, E. (1982). The assessment and significance of habituation to a repeated stimulus by the human fetus. Early Human Development, 7, 211-219.

Leader, L. R., & Bennett, M. J. (1988). Fetal habituation. In M. I. Levene, M. J. Bennett, & J. Punt (Eds.),Fetal and neonatal neurology and neurosurgery (pp.59-70). Edinburgh, Scotland: Churchill.

Lecaunet, J-P., Fifer, W.P., Krasnegor, N.A. & Smotherman, W.P. Eds. (1995). Fetal Development: A Psychobiological Perspective, Erlbaum:New Jersey.
Leifer, M. (1980). Psychological effects of motherhood. New York: Prager.
Lewis, M & Brooks-Gunn, J. (1981) Visual attention as a predictor of cognitive function at two years of age. Intelligence, 5, 131-140.
Lagercrantz, H., & Bistoletti, P. (1977). Catecholamine release in the newborn. Pediatric Research, 11, 889-893.
Lagercrantz, H., & Slotkin, T. A., (1986). The "stress" of being born. Scientific American, 254,100 107.
Lecanuet, J., Granier-Deferre, C., & Busnel, M. (1989). Differential fetal auditory reactiveness as a function of stimulus characteristics and state. Seminars in Perinatology, 13(5), 421-429.
Leon, M. (1992). The neurobiology of filial learning. Annual Review of Psychology, 43, 377-98.
Liggins, G. C. (1982). The fetus and birth. In C. R. Austin & R. V. Short (Eds.), Reproduction in mammals, Book 2: Embryonic and fetal development (pp. 114-141). New York: Cambridge University Press.
Martin, C. B. (1981). Behavioral states in the human fetus. The Journal of Reproductive Medicine, 26, 425-432.
Manders, M. A. et al (1997). The effects of maternal exercise on fetal heart rate and movement patterns. Early Human Development, 48, 237-247.
Maurer, D. (1985). Infants' perception of facedness. In T.N. Field & N. Fox (Eds.), Social-Perception in Infants. Norwood, NJ: Ablex.
Maurer, D. & Young, R. (1983). Newborn's following of natural and distorted arrangements of facial features. Infant Behav & Development, 6, 127-131.
McCall, R. B. (1981) Early predictors of later IQ: The search continues. Intelligence, 5, 141-147.
Meltzoff, A. N. & Moore, M. K. (1977). Imitation of facial and manual gestures by human neonates. Science, 198, 75-78.
Meltzoff, A. N. & Borton, R. W. (1979) Intermodal matching by human neonates. Nature, 282, 403-404.
Michel, G.F., Harkins, D.A. & Meserve, A.L. (1990). Sex differences in neonatal state and lateralized head orientation. Infant Behavior and Development, 13, 461-467.
Moon, C., Cooper, R. P., & Fifer, W. P. (1993). Two-day-olds prefer their native language. Infant Behavior and Development, 16(4), 495-500.
Moon, C., & Fifer, W. (1990). Syllables as signals for 2-day-old infants. Infant Behavior and Development, 13, 377-390.
Moore, K.L. (1982) The Developing Fetus: Clinically Oriented Embryology. Philadelphia:WB Saunders.
Muller, M. E. (1993). Development of a prenatal attachment inventory. Western Journal of Nursing Research, 15, 199-215.
Muller, M. E. (1996). Prenatal and postnatal attachment: a modest correlation. Journal of Obstetrics, Gynecology & Neonatal Nursing, 25, 161-166.
Nagy, E. (2001). Gender-related differences in rectal temperature in human neonates. Early Human Development, 64, 37-43.
Narayanan, C. H., Fox, M. W., & Hamburger, V. (1971). Prenatal development of spontaneous and evoked activity in the rat. Behavior, 40,100-134.
Nijhuis, J. G. (1986). Behavioural states: Concomitants, clinical implications and the assessment of the condition of the nervous system. European Journal of Obstetrics and Gynecology and Reproductive Biology, 21, 301-308.
Nishimura, H. (1977) Prenatal development of the human: An atlas. National Institutes of Health: Washington DC.
Nishimura, H. (1983). Atlas of Prenatal Histology. Igaku-Shoin, Tokyo.

O'Rahilly, R. and Muller, F. (1994). The embryonic human brain: An atlas of developmental stages. New York: Wiley-Liss.
Ohta, M. (1987). Cognitive disorders of infantile autism: A study employing the WISC, spatial relationship conceptualization, and gesture imitations. Journal of Autism and Developmental Disorders, 17,45-62.
Oster, H. (1978). Facial expression and affect development. In M. Lewis and L. A. Rosenblum (eds.), The development of affect. New York: Plenum.
Oyama, S. (1985). The ontogeny of information: Developmental systems and information. New York: Cambridge University Press.
Page, E. W., Villee, C. A., & Villee, D. B. (1981). Human reproduction: Essentials of reproductive and perinatal medicine. Philadelphia: W. B. Saunders.
Papousek, M. and Papousek, H. (1981). Musical elements in the infants vocalization: their significance for communication, cognition and creativity. In L. P. Lipsitt and C. K. Rovee-Collier (eds.), Advances in infancy research, vol. 1. Norwood, NJ: Ablex.
Papousek, M., Papousek, H. and Harris, B. J. (1987). The emergence of play in parent-infant interactions. In D. Gorlitz and J. F. Wohlwill (eds.), Curiosity, imagination and play: On the development of spontaneous cognitive and motivational processes (pp.214-46). Hillsdale, NJ: Erlbaum
Parry, M. H. (1972). Infants'responses to novelty in familiar and unfamiliar settings. Child Development, 43, 233-237.
Pedersen, P. E., & Blass, E. M. (1982). Prenatal & postnatal determinants of the first suckling episode in albino rats. Dev. Psychobiology, 15, 349-355.
Peiper, A. (1925). Sinnesempfindungen des Kindes vor seiner geburt [The sensory awareness of the child before birth]. Monatsschriftfur Kinderheilkunde, 29, 237-241.
Pena, M., Birch, D., Uauy, R & Peirano, P. (1999). The effect of sleep state on electroretinographic (ERG) activity during early human development. Early Human Development, 55, 51-62.
Phillips, R.D., Wagner, S. H., Fells, C.A. & Lynch, M. (1990). Do infants recognize emotion in facial expressions? Infant Behavior and Development, 13, 71-84.
Pike, A.A., Marlow, N. & Reber, C. (1999). Maturation of flash visual evoked potential in preterm infants. Early Human Development, 54, 215-222.
Pomerleau-Malcuit, A., & Clifton, R. K. (1973). Neonatal heart-rate response to tactile, auditory, and vestibular stimulation in different states. Child Development, 44, 485-496.
Porac, C., & Coren, S. (1981). Lateral preferences and human behavior. New York: Springer-Verlag.
Previc, F. (1991). A general theory concerning the prenatal origins of cerebral lateralization in humans. Psychological Review, 98, 299-334.
Pujol, R., Lavigne-Rebillard, M., & Uziel, A. (1990). Physiological correlates of development of human cochlea. Seminars in Perinatology, 14, 275-280.
Querleu, D., Renard, X., Boutteville, C., & Crepin, G. (1989). Hearing by the human fetus? Seminars in Perinatology, 13(5), 409-420.
Rafal, R.D., Henick, A., & Smith, J. (1991). Extrageniculate contribution to reflex visual orienting in normal humans: a temporal hemifield advantage. Journal of Cognitive Neuroscience, 3, 351-358.
Reynolds, S. R. M. (1962). Nature of fetal adaptation to the uterine environment: A problem of sensory deprivation. American Journal of Obstetrics and Gynecology, 83, 800-808.
Ronca, A. E., & Alberts, J. R. (1990). Heart rate development and sensory-evoked cardiac responses in perinatal rats. Physiology & Behavior, 47, 1075-1082.
Ronca, A. E., & Alberts, J. R. (1994). Sensory stimuli associated with gestation and parturition evoke cardiac and behavioral responses in fetal rats. Psychobiology 55, 270-282.

Ronca, A. E., Lamkin, C. A., & Alberts, J. R. (1993). Maternal contributions to sensory experience in the fetal and newborn rat (Rattus norvegicus). Journal of Comparative Psychology, 107, 61-74.
Rosenblatt, J. S. (1963). Maternal behavior in the laboratory rat. In H. L. Rheingold (Ed.), Maternal behavior in mammals. New York: Wiley.
Salk, L. (1962) Mothers' heartbeat as an imprinting stimulus. Transactions of the New York Academy of Science, 24, 753-763.
Salvador, H. S. & Koos, B. J. (1989). Effects of regular and decaffeinated coffee on fetal breathing and heart rate. American Journal of Obstetrics and Gynecology, 160, 1043-1047.
Scarpelli, E. M., Condorelli, S., & Cosmi, E. V. (1977). Cutaneous stimulation and generation of breathing in the fetus. Pediatric Research, 11, 24-28.
Segalowitz, S. J., & Bryden, M. P. (1983). Individual differences in hemisperic representation of language. In S. J. Segalowitz (Ed.), Languagefunctions and brain organization (pp. 341-372). New York: Academic Press
Seidler, F., & Slotkin, T. A. (1985). Adrenomedullary function in the neonatal rat: Responses to acute hypoxia. Journal of Physiology, 358, 1-16.
Shahidullah, S., & Hepper, P. G. (1992). Abnormal fetal behaviour in first trimester spontaneous abortion. European Journal of Obstetrics, Gynecology and Reproductive Biology, 45,181-184.
Siddiqui, A, & Hagglof, B. (2000). Does maternal prenatal attachment predict postnatal mother-infant interaction? Early Human Development, 59, 13-25.
Silver, M., & Edwards, A. V. (1980). The development of the sympatho-adrenal system with an assessment of the role of the adrenal medulla in the fetus and newborn. In H. Parvez & S. Parvez (Eds.), Biogenic amines in development (pp. 147-212). New York: Elsevier Biomedical Press.
Simion, F., Valenza, E., Umilta, C., & Dalla Barba, B. (1998). Preferential orienting to faces in newborns: a temporal-nasal asymmetry. Journal of Experimental Psychology (Human Perception and Performance), 76, 45-56.
Simion, F, Valenza, E & Umilta, C (1998). Mechanisms underlying face preference at birth. In Simion, F and Butterworth, G. (Eds.), The Development of Sensory, Motor and Cognitive Capacities in Early Infancy: From Perception to Cognition, Psychology Press, pp 87-102.
Slater, A. et al (1998). Newborn infants prefer attractive faces. Infant Behavior and Development, 21, 345-354.
Slater, A. (1993). Visual perceptual abilities at birth: implications for face perception. In B. de Boysson-Bardies et al. (Eds.), Developmental Neurocognition:Face Processing in the First Year of Life. New York: Academic
Slater, A.M., Earle, D.C., Morison, V., & Rose, D. (1985). Pattern preferences at birth and their interaction with habituation induced novelty preferences. Journal of Experimental Child Psychology, 39, 37-54.
Slater, A., Morison, V., & Somers, M. (1988). Orientation discrimination and cortical function in the human newborn. Perception, 17, 596-602.
Slater A. (Ed.) (1998). Perceptual Development: Visual, auditory and speech perception in infancy. Psychology Press:New York
Smotherman, W. P. (1982). Odor aversion learning by the rat fetus. Physiology & Behavior, 29, 769-771.
Sokol, R. J. & Rosen, M. G. (1974). The fetal electroencephalogram. Clinics in Obstetrics and Gynaecology, 1, 123-138.
Spence, M. J., & DeCasper, A. J. (1987). Prenatal experience with low-frequency maternal-voice sounds influences neonatal perception of maternal voice samples. Infant Behavior and Development, 16, 133-142.
St. James-Roberts, I & Menon-Johansson, P. (1999). Predicting infant crying from fetal movement data. Early Human Development, 54, 55-62.

Storm, H. (2001). Development of emotional sweating in preterms measured by skin conductance changes. Early Human Development, 62, 149-158.

Streeter, G. L. (1920). Weight, sitting height, head size, foot length, and menstrual age of the human embryo. Contributions to Embryology of Carnegie Institute, 111, 143-170.

Streeter, G. L. (1951). Developmental horizons in human embryos. Age groups XI to XXIII. Carnegie Institution of Washington. Washington DC.

Thompson, R. F., & Spencer, W. A. (1966). Habituation: A model for the study of neuronal substrates of behavior. Psychological Review, 73,16-43.

Trevarthan, C. Kokkinaki, T. & Fiamenghi, G. A. (1999). What infants' imitations communicate: with mothers, with fathers and with peers. In J. Nadel & G. Butterworth (Eds.), Imitation in Infancy. Cambridge Univ. Press:Cambridge.

Valenza, E., Simion, F., Macchi Cassia, V., & Umilta, C. (1996). Face preference at birth. Journal of Experimental Psychology: Human Perception and Performance, 27, 892-903.

van Heteren, C. F., Boekkooi, P. F., Jongsma, H. W. & Nijhuis, J. G. (2001). Fetal habituation to vibroacoustic stimulation in relation to fetal states and fetal heart rate parameters. Early Human Development, 61, 135-145.

Varendi, H., Christensson, K, Porter, R. H. & Winberg, J. (1998). Soothing effect of amniotic fluid smell in newborn infants. Early Human Development, 51, 47-55.

Ververs, I.A., Van-Gelder, M.R., DeVries, J.I., Hopkins, B & Van Geijn, H.P. (1998). Prenatal development of arm posture. Early Human Development, 51, 61-70.

Witelson, S. F., & Paille, W. (1973). Left hemisphere specialisation for language in the newborn: Neuroanatomical evidence of asymmetry. Brain, 96, 641- 646.

Worthington-Roberts, B. (1996). Nutrition in Pregnancy and Lactation. McGraw-hill: New York.

Yin, R.H. (1969). Looking at upside-down faces. Journal of Experimental Psychology, 81, 141-145.

Yin, R.H. (1978). The parietal lobe and visual attention. Journal of Psychiatric Research, 14,261-266.

Zimmer, E. Z., Chao, C. R., Guy, G. P., Marks, F., & Fifer, W. P. (1993). Vibroacoustic stimulation evokes human fetal micturition. Obstetrics and Gynecology, S1(2), 178-180.

Zimmer, E. Z., Fifer, W. P., Kim, Y., Rey, H. R., Chao, C. R., & Myers, M. M. (1993). Response of the premature fetus to stimulation by speech sounds. Early Human Development, 33, 207-215.

For the latest information on Becoming a Baby, please visit our web site at BecomingaBaby.com

Enjoy your new baby!